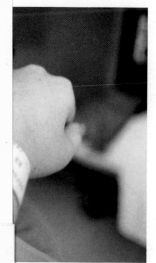

the
C
Word

The C-Word

Teenagers and Their Families Living with Cancer

by Elena Dorfman

Foreword by John T. Truman, M.D.

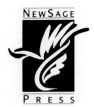

NewSage Press

**To my mother, Virginia, and to George, my uncle,
who are always with me.**

**The C-Word: Teenagers and Their Families
Living with Cancer**

Address inquiries to NewSage Press
825 N.E. 20th Avenue, Suite 150
Portland, OR 97232

First Edition 1994

Designed by Ed Marquand
Printed in Korea through Print Vision,
Portland, Oregon

Library of Congress
Cataloging-in-Publication Data

Dorfman, Elena, 1965
    The C-word : teenagers and their fami-
lies living with cancer / by Elena Dorfman :
foreword by John T. Truman, Md.
        p.   cm.
    Includes bibliographical references.
    ISBN 0-939165-21-X : $16.95
    1. Tumors in adolescence. [1. Cancer—
Patients.]   I. Title.

RC281.C4D67 1994
362.1'96994'00835—dc20   93-32041
                                 CIP
                                 AC

Acknowledgments

In the four years I spent working on this book, I encountered many people who supported and encouraged me. I would like to be able to thank everyone, but most importantly my deepest gratitude goes to the individual teenagers and their families who opened up their hearts and homes to me. This book would have been impossible to complete without their trust and belief in the project.

I am grateful to the following doctors and care-givers on whom I depended for introductions and entrance into their hospitals: Margaret Adams Greenly and the staff of Memorial Sloan-Kettering Cancer Center; Dr. Donald Medearis and Dr. William Ferguson and the staff of Massachusetts General Hospital; Rachael Goldsborough and the oncology department of Children's Hospital Oakland; and Dr. Carol Diamond and the staff of the pediatric oncology department of Kaiser Permanente, San Francisco. I would also like to acknowledge the staff of Massachusetts General Hospital who cared for me when I was ill. Their patience, love, humor, and understanding remain with me to this day.

Others I wish to thank for their continuous support include: Joan Harrison, Joan Marks, James Tulsky, Ilana Saraf, Louise Franklin, Mark Dowie, Ava and Susan Abramowitz, Tammi Montier, Michelle Bruton, Justin Sullivan, Julie Queen, Paul Lundahl, Eric Ladenberg, Barbara Tropp, and Kirk Anspach, who printed my photographs. A special thanks to my editors and publishers, Maureen Michelson and Rhonda Hughes, who have shown me and this work tremendous sensitivity and respect.

For their interest and encouragement, I am grateful to the following members of my family: Ira, Marilyn, Arthur, Sandra, Catherine, Martin, and Dorothy. I would also like to thank Dore Gardner for her friendship, advice, and thoughtfulness; Susan Jahoda, who helped uncover my passion for this idea and set the wheels in motion; Carolyn Moore, who generously contributed her insights and ideas; Eugene Richards, for his initial enthusiasm and advice; and Bill Burke, for asking me, during a discouraging period, what else I had to do with my time that was as important.

Elena Dorfman

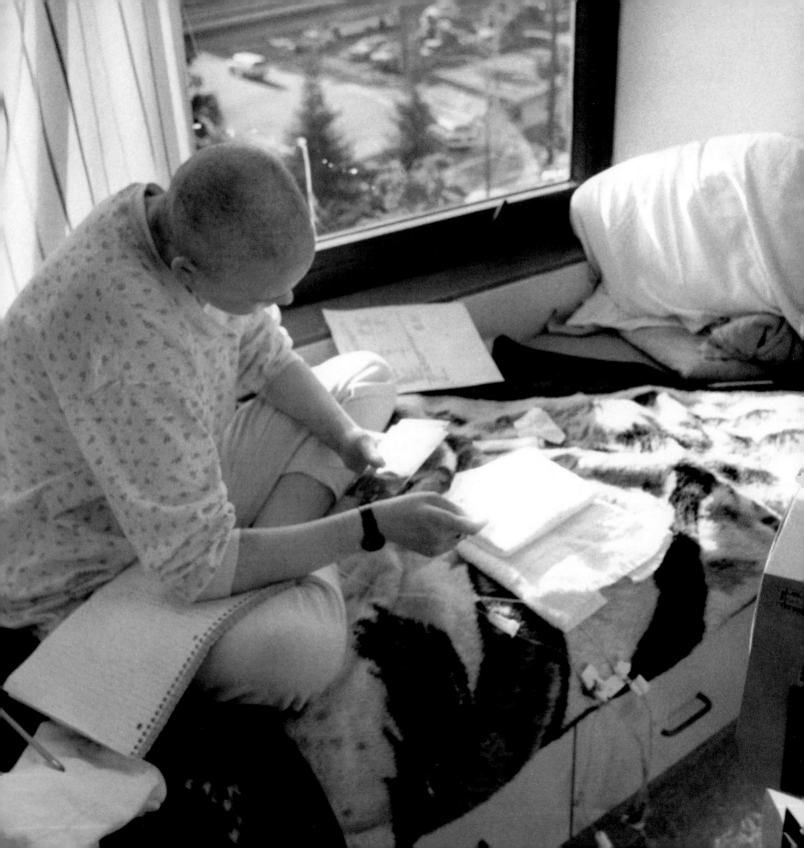

Contents

Foreword

This wonderful book tells us much about life. Through the eyes of young people we learn how precious yet how fragile it is. Perhaps only after confronting the imminent prospect of death can we truly appreciate the beauty of life. The words of these patients and families can act as a substitute for those of us who have yet to face death personally. If their words force us to consider how we should react when our time comes, then this book will have served a very useful purpose. If their words inspire us to face our future with the optimism, determination, and strength with which these young people have faced theirs, then we will owe an incalculable debt of gratitude to the subjects of this book and to its author.

Cancer in young people under age 21 is quite different from cancer in adults. For one thing, there are virtually no carcinomas such as lung, bowel, breast, pancreas, or prostate. The commonest childhood cancer is leukemia. Then, in descending order of frequency, come brain tumors, Wilms' tumor of the kidney, neuroblastoma, rhabdomyosarcoma, and the bone tumors. When I started looking after children with cancer thirty years ago, the overall cure rate was dismal. Every child with leukemia died, and cure was unheard of. Most children with brain tumors, the lymphomas, neuroblastoma, rhabdomyosarcoma, and the bone tumors died. Only those with Wilms' tumor had any real chance of cure.

By the early '70s, there was much more hope for cure in most of these tumors, largely as a result of more effective chemotherapy. By the mid-'80s it was clear that we were winning in a vast majority of these areas. Now, in the '90s, we fully expect that at least two out of three children with cancer will outlive their doctors and be truly cured of their cancer. Unfortunately, the treatment is long and arduous, with many predictable and unpredictable side effects. To many children, the treatment seems worse than the disease. During the difficult teenage years, the problems of adolescence are greatly intensified by the knowledge that the individual has cancer and may die from it. And the side effects of treatment compound the difficulties.

Let me tell you about a teenage patient I treated about ten years ago. Out of the blue she found out that she had rhabdomyosarcoma, a cancer of the muscle tissue, the cause of which is unknown, and which occurs in fewer than one thousand Americans each year. She would need to have surgery and radiation therapy, and then, worst of all, two full years of chemotherapy. That was where I came in, it being my job as a pediatric oncologist to administer the chemotherapy. She was very upset about having cancer in the first place, and although she could understand the need for surgery and radiation therapy, the chemotherapy was a different matter. The side effects would be dreadful. The chemotherapy was to go on for two long years, and it was not so obvious why that was necessary if the tumor seemed to have been eradicated from its original location. Reluctantly, she went along with her family and with me and started the chemotherapy.

The side effects were indeed unpleasant. She lost all her hair, had severe nausea and vomiting, bad aches and pains, mouth sores, and numbness of fingers and toes. Once when she was in the hospital getting chemotherapy I brought in a high-school volunteer who didn't even recognize her as her tentmate at the summer camp the year before. Yet the patient knew that the alternative was death and that she had to undergo chemotherapy even though she didn't like it. She was very angry, at fate for having singled her out to have cancer, and at her doctors for giving her treatment that was so unpleasant. Intellectually she understood perfectly well why she needed each treatment, but that didn't mean she had to like it, or accept it without complaint.

One thing she quickly learned was how concerned everyone became when she lost weight after a particularly nauseating session of chemotherapy. This became a very useful weapon to indicate how unpleasant she found the chemotherapy, and perhaps to make everyone feel guilty as well. When she was threatened with a feeding tube if she didn't weigh ninety-five pounds at her next weigh-in, she would arrange to weigh exactly ninety-five pounds. Afterward she would starve herself back to eighty-seven pounds, and everyone would become apprehensive again. However, she never allowed her weight to interfere with the actual timing or dosages; she was much too intelligent for that.

Several years afterward, when all the unpleasantness had passed and it was obvious that she was cured, she told me how powerless she felt during the treatment and how she had used her anorexia to exercise what little control she had left. She told me how important it had been for her that everyone had listened to her and been honest with her about everything that was about to happen. She also told me how grateful she was that all her doctors and nurses had let her act out her emotions without holding it against her and that she had felt safe in the clinic expressing her innermost feelings. I told her that no patient had ever frustrated or angered us more than she because she knew exactly what our concerns were and played on them at all times. Still, we both respected each other's position even during the worst of times. She knew that I had to do what I was doing because it was in her best interest, and I knew that she had to act out as she was because it was in her nature to give honest expression to her feelings.

It is thus a very great honor for me to write the foreword to this book because Elena Dorfman was this patient. If anyone knows the value of life, it is Elena. If anyone knows the importance of fighting the good fight, it is Elena. If anyone knows the power of emotions, it is Elena. And if anyone can capture in print the eternal goodness of the human spirit in the face of adversity, it is Elena.

John T. Truman, M.D.

Introduction

When I was 16 I found a lump in my left wrist that, when left alone, grew to the size of a large marble. I was told I had tendinitis but late in my junior year of high school was diagnosed with rhabdomyosarcoma, cancer of the soft tissue. On the same day as my diagnosis, my mother was told that the lump she had found in her breast was malignant.

It was and still is unfathomable to try to understand how my mother and I could both have cancer at the same time. We were dispirited and worried and overly protective of each other. Our relationship turned abrupt and often explosive. I know that much of what I experienced was magnified by our concurrent illnesses. Together, over time, we learned to deal with the stresses, and prior to my mother's death, we became closer than we ever had been before.

In the beginning, I became angry at everything. I threw chairs at the doctors when they told me what chemotherapy was and what to expect as side effects. I didn't want to lose my hair. I didn't want to throw up. I didn't want to have to ask permission to go out of town, and if granted, leave with a list of instructions and the drugs I was taking. I didn't want to lose my arm. The changes in me were fast and extreme, and I didn't recognize myself anymore. I was gaunt and bald. My skin took on a yellowish tone. I was scared. My body had let something poisonous grow inside me. I felt betrayed.

It was agonizing to confront the hospital, the huge gray building, my second home, knowing my friends could continue to lead their normal lives. They could date, go to the movies, eat Chinese food and ice cream. That's all I could think of during my five days of constant nausea, every three weeks, for the twenty-six months in which I followed my chemotherapy like a recipe: cytoxan, adriamycin, vincristine. For good measure, radiation was also thrown in. Small tattooed Xs were the boundaries of the rays that killed the bad cells, and a guard was made to protect my increasingly brittle wrist.

I remember very well the strange-tasting fluid that gathered under my jawbone when I walked into the hospital. I remember the sour smell of the hand lotion they gave out—one that I could never use at home. I remember the long, cold, curved needle that injected the medicines

11

through my Port-a-Cath (vein implant). I remember the bone marrow tests, the searching in head, hands, and feet for fresh veins, the X rays, the three A.M. weigh-ins, and the dull, strange sleep I would slip into as a result of the antinausea drugs. At the time, I thought it would never end. But it did. And I have been told by my oncologists not to return for check-ups. I do not need them anymore.

When I was ill, I desperately needed a person, or a book, that I could identify with. My family and a few very close friends were supportive and encouraging, but I felt their understanding was limited. I wanted to know what a 17-year-old girl looked like without hair and where she went to find a wig. I wanted to know how others handled a low self-image, hard to ignore with the vast change in appearance. And I wanted to know how someone else reacted when a friend or roommate or fellow chemo patient died. I needed to feel I was not the only one in the world going through such changes. I wanted to look at something that would lessen the isolation I felt and take me beyond the superficial, clinical manner of a hospital pamphlet. Several years later, when I was in college, I was encouraged to pursue an idea I'd had to photograph teenagers with cancer.

This book is an attempt to make sense of my illness by combining pictures and personal experiences of young adults facing cancer today. They are working through the normal difficulties of being teenagers, years made much more complex by the onset of cancer. As each of these teenagers expressed, when you are sick, it is hard not to feel that the world is spinning by without you. I hope the experiences of these young people will provide deep inspiration to the readers of this book.

> Last night I dreamt someone leaned close
> and whispered, "Who told you it would
> ever be over? How could you think you
> would ever get away with living?" I was
> lying on my back with tubes sticking down
> my nose and throat. A knife was digging
> into the malignant lumps that had grown
> inside me. My cancer had recurred.

These dreams that I have and the fears of a recurrence may never leave me, but I do not regret my intimacy with illness. It has brought me far beyond the place I was before I knew this disease. This piece of work is my gift in return. The completion of this book will close my ten-year chapter with cancer. I am certain that no other endeavor I undertake will be as personal or as close to my heart.

Elena Dorfman

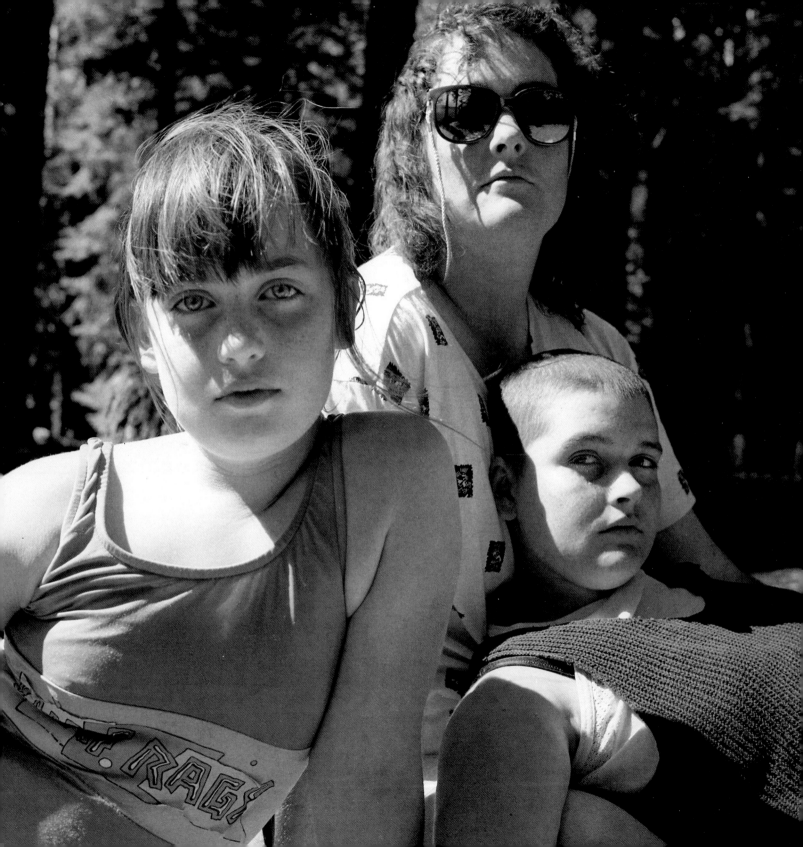

Jennifer

16 years old
Acute lymphoblastic leukemia

Jennifer has been getting chemotherapy treatment for acute lymphoblastic leukemia for five months when I first meet her. She lives with her family in Klamath Falls, Oregon, but travels to Children's Hospital Oakland, in California for her cancer treatments.

Over the course of the two years that we know each other, Jenny, her family, and I are in frequent contact. During that time, she has many setbacks, sometimes quarantined in the hospital for up to six weeks at a time due to high fevers and infections in her mouth. Although her cancer treatments involve extended periods of time spent alone and painful medical procedures, Jenny maintains her ability to laugh and find faith within herself. I think much of the confidence she conjures up is due to the constant attention and devotion from her mother, Vicki, and her father, Greg.

At the time of our first interview, Jenny, her parents, and two younger sisters are staying in San Francisco at the home of the children's great-grandmother, while Jenny receives outpatient treatment at the hospital.

March 1991

Jenny
Vicki, Jennifer's mother

How did you find out you had cancer?

Jenny: We went to the doctor because I had one swollen lymph node behind my ear. I thought it was a spider bite or something. The doctor told us to try some dandruff shampoo. I had a lot of pain in my bones, my liver, and spleen. Two days later they kicked me out of school because they thought I had the mumps. I was really sick by the time we saw the

Jenny (right) with her mother, Vicki, and sister Joanna.

second doctor. He was 99 percent sure it was the mumps but wanted to do a test. A few days later they called us to say the mumps test was negative, and he was beginning to suspect something serious.

At that point we decided not to deal with the hospital in Oregon, which is near where we live, but rather to go to Children's Hospital in the Bay Area. We'd dealt with them before, and we have family down there. We grabbed some clothes and traveled all day to get to the hospital. I was in a wheelchair and looking so sick that they almost didn't let me on the plane. That was on a Thursday.

I was diagnosed on Friday and had my bone marrow test and started chemotherapy immediately. I had to take prednisone, daunomycin, vincristine, and asparginase. At one time, I was taking over twenty pills a day, plus antibiotics. For the first four or five days, they kept me in isolation. I stayed in the hospital about ten days in all. My weight went from 107 to 118 pounds. Some days I was ordering three trays of food at a time. The prednisone was making me really hungry!

Vicki: The prednisone also caused a lot of mood swings. I don't think Jenny recognized that when it was happening. And when her hemoglobin got low, she would get really exhausted. Then she'd have a transfusion and feel better. It took us a few days to realize where these changes were coming from.

Jenny: We had a couple of really fun nights in the hospital. Especially "the night from hell," as we like to call it. It had to do with a tube that went up my nose, down my throat, and into my stomach. They wanted me to drink seven cups of potassium, but I couldn't keep it down. I was up all night with the nurses pouring it down my throat. My blood sugar went up to around 400. I ended up having to be on a diabetic diet for a while.

Were you frightened by all of this?

Jenny: No, I was usually really loaded on painkillers and antinausea medicine. I could barely open my eyes I was so tired. I loved the Demerol [painkiller]. I would say all kinds of crazy things when I was on it.

Vicki: When Jenny was wheeled in for her bone marrow test, she kept saying, "I really want to tell some jokes, but I can't remember any."

Jenny: A psychologist visited me while I was in the hospital. I think I really intimidated her. I didn't mean to, but I just didn't feel I needed her. If I want to talk to someone, I have other people to talk to—friends and family.

When I found out I had cancer, it all happened so quickly in the beginning. We didn't even have time to tell the school. Nobody, not even my friends, knew what had happened. I told my teacher a few weeks later, and he told the rest of the school. A lot of them wrote letters and sent cards. I've been out of school for three months, and it's been announced on the intercom almost every day. The school, and the theater in town, had a few benefits for me. I've had kids from other schools calling me to tell me about their experiences with being sick. I went to the basketball team and thanked them for their cards. They asked me questions about being sick, and when I left, they gave me a standing ovation.

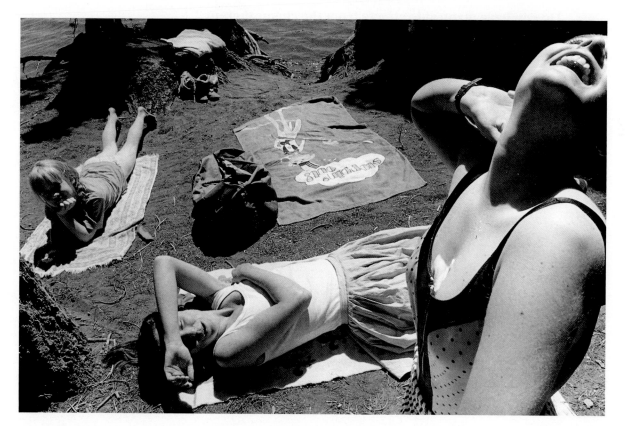

Jenny (right) at the beach with her family.

17

Do your sisters and brother understand your illness?

Jenny: They are all super smart. My youngest sister wrote a paper about my being sick that was published in the hospital newsletter. Her class wrote me letters while I was in the hospital, and when I got home my sister took me to her class for show and tell.

How did it feel when you lost your hair?

Jenny: I had waist-length hair. I knew I was going to lose it. First we cut it above my ears. Going bald after that wasn't so bad. It was funny because when I first went into a store, everybody was trying hard not to look at me, but I could see them peeking the whole time. Now I walk around school without anything on my head. Wigs are so scratchy. I keep losing my eyebrows and eyelashes. Why don't I lose the hair on my legs or under my arms, where I want to?

Do you have many side effects from the chemotherapy?

Jenny: For a while I shook really bad. The vincristine affects my muscle coordination, so it's hard to walk up stairs. My school is four stories high, and I have lots of climbing there. And when I'm off the vincristine, I get charley horses in my hands and legs. My hands get disfigured from them. And I've had really bad mouth sores from the methotrexate. I told them in the hospital that I don't want to know about possible side effects. Just do it and let me be.

I went to one of the teen support groups they offered. I was on prednisone, and I went for the pizza. I told jokes and ate half a pizza. I was the only teen there. Everyone was under 11. In the hospital teen room, I was always the only teen there. I didn't have access to anyone my age in the world who had cancer and is alive.

Vicki: I've had a hard time finding books with any real information on cancer. There was a library at the hospital, but it was only open to the doctors. I had to look covertly for titles and get a nurse to check them out. The doctors said they would answer any questions I had, but I can't even begin to formulate a question if I don't have more than the surface material. I've been sort of the keeper of my children's health all these years. This cancer is something out of my league, but the more I know, the more I can protect Jenny.

Fortunately, there is an oncologist coming to our local hospital this summer. There are many children here with cancer, but they all go out of the area for treatment. We live in Oregon but go to Children's Hospital in California. And that gets difficult because the insurance company wants to pay Oregon rural rates. But it's the incidental costs that are almost harder than the medical costs: traveling, food, medicine. A little bottle of pills costs sixty dollars. Jenny is aware of the burden of these costs, and I'm sure it is a burden for her too, even if it's not spoken.

We don't really feel like we have any handle on what's going on with the medical costs. The insurance company will pay 90 percent for one treatment and 10 percent for another. Why? Which treatment is right and which one is wrong? It's not like this is a car we're talking about, where we can try a used alternator first and if that doesn't work, then we'll get a new one. We're talking about Jenny, a human being. You really have to shop around and do research to know what you're buying in health insurance. But most people aren't counting on having a cata-strophic illness.

As consumers, there is no sense of power for us in the "hallowed halls" of the hospital. When I'm there, I can't say, "Excuse me, Jenny's going to be discharged in fifteen minutes, so maybe this isn't a good time to start that IV." There are schedules and procedures, and it's all very automatic. And to question any of that, you risk looking like a par-ent who's not valuing your child's well-being.

Jenny: I've had some pretty bad experiences. The worst was probably when I had to have a bone marrow test at a hospital in Klamath Falls [Oregon]. Two pathologists had to do it, and I don't think they'd ever done one before. They had to take a bone sample twice, and we were there for at least an hour while they were tearing into my back. The inci-sion was oozing for days, and it was really painful and sore. I had never cried, but that time I cried and cried and cried. I'm not going back there again.

How long will you be getting treatments?

Jenny: About two and a half years. Feels like forever now. I've already been through phases one through four in my chemotherapy treatment. After the first six months of these drugs, I'll be on a maintenance schedule that isn't as intense. I can probably get those drugs at home and just come down to Children's Hospital in California for periodic checkups. I don't know what's going to happen with me. A few months ago I was around a lot of death. An old boyfriend died in a car crash. My friend and her mom *both* died of cancer. And another friend was diagnosed with leukemia. And then I was diagnosed. It happens. Good things can come of it. I haven't asked, "Why me?" You do what you can and that's it.

April 1991

One month after my first meeting with Jenny and her mother, Jenny has a very serious reaction to her chemotherapy drugs that results in life threatening seizures. While hospitalized for the seizures, Jenny develops horrendous mouth sores that keep her bedridden, unable to eat or speak, for several weeks.

Jenny has to be transported by air ambulance from the hospital in Oregon to Children's Hospital in California. Jenny's mother, Vicki, is staying with her in California while Jenny's father, Greg, stays home with the other three children. Vicki and I talk alone for a long time one afternoon while Jenny is resting in her hospital room.

Vicki, Jenny's mother

Jenny showing her Broviac vein implant.

I want people to know there is more to life than leukemia, even during this. It's hard for us both when she's in the hospital because I feel reduced to one subject. I hate that. But there is more to our lives than this.

I hope Jenny sees that Greg and I are here for her. She doesn't have to go through this on her own. I've seen the relationship between Jenny and her father change so much. I hope she sees that he'll drop everything and come in a minute to help her. I think you have a relationship your whole life with your kids where you are there for them, and they don't always see it.

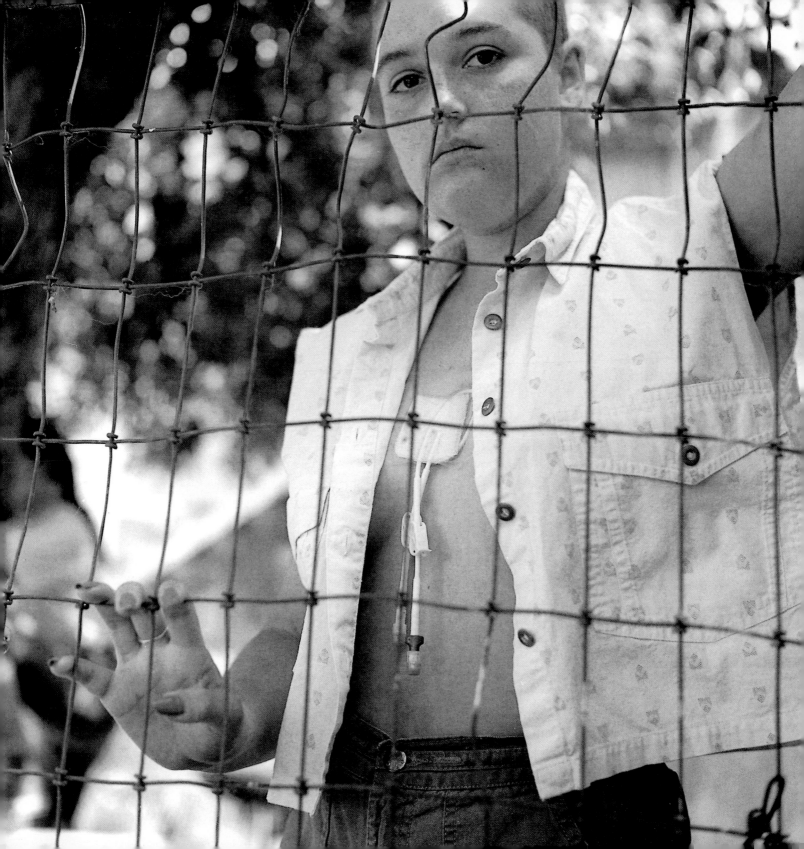

I would say that Jenny is already a better person. Maybe not better, but she has grown in these past six months so much. It's my nature to look at the bright side of things. There was a new family on the oncology floor last week. The daughter was diagnosed a couple days before, and the parents were so overwhelmed. I told them, "Through all of this you will find hidden blessings." I also told them that nothing is etched in stone, and they shouldn't put anything on their calendar that can't be changed.

I hope Jenny sees that there are people who are there for us. For example, someone called me last week about this event called the Benefit Bowl. The National Guard base and the state police get together for a series of events to raise money for one family who is in need. Someone gave them our name, and they wanted us to come in for an interview. We went and talked for forty-five minutes to some representatives for Benefit Bowl. They asked us questions and told us they would talk about it and get back to us in a couple of weeks. They called Greg that night and said that they had unanimously chosen our family.

At the end of this month there will be a concert at the theater in town. And various little events will go on between now and November to raise money for Jenny's treatments. I heard someone say that you need to make friends before you need them. It just struck me as being so true. But Jenny's old enough that she's just got to be herself. I want her to be perfect—I'm her mother. I don't want her to be snippy with a nurse. I want her to say, "Thank you for my medicine!"

I see that Jenny doesn't always acknowledge when she's doing better. People will come into the room and say, "You look so much better than you did last week." She'll say, "I don't feel better at all." I think it's because Jenny's afraid that we'll all think, "Well, OK, you should be fine now, see you later." I don't know. I have tried to say to Jenny, "I know your mouth still really hurts from all the sores, but I'm glad you're looking better and your body is responding well to the medication." Right now all she can see are the limitations and the pain of her disease.

I remember the first time Jenny was discharged from the hospital. It was like cutting the umbilical cord. I wished the whole hospital could come home with me. My friend Judith, who has a 5-year-old with leukemia, stayed in the hospital three extra days because she was too scared to go home. At least in the hospital they know what's going on. We really felt this when we came back to Children's Hospital after her seizures in Oregon. It was almost like a physical sigh of relief when we got here.

At Children's Hospital you get a team of oncologists. Whoever is on the floor is who you get. Whoever is in the clinic is who you get. It really doesn't matter. You find that, knowing how the different doctors respond, you might save your question for next week when you know a certain doctor might be on. When there is a team, none of them feels like your doctor. I think that's what I'm going to like about the new oncologist at home in Klamath Falls. It meant a lot to me that the doctor in Klamath Falls kept calling us at the hospital. She didn't call Jenny's doctor in California to get his opinion, she called me.

The only down side of this is that the doctor doesn't have a pediatric oncology staff to support her, which makes a huge difference. The hospital Jenny uses is just the hospital in the community, it's not a children's hospital. If Jenny were on the oncology floor, she'd be with geriatric patients. Before, I would have preferred a general pediatric floor, but now I prefer an oncology floor. I think the medical staff are more cognizant of the heightened susceptibility to infection. I don't think Jenny's mouth sores would have gotten this bad if we had been treated here in time. They weren't aggressive about treatments or medicine. On an oncology floor, they know what to look for.

A few days ago Jenny was able to eat a lot. She took in about 1,500 calories each day. Then some new sores came up, and she cut way back again. The medicine keeps Jenny's weight up, which she doesn't like. I don't think she looks at the fact that there is more to it than just weight. It really is about protein and nutrition. Jenny's afraid to go home, to go back to the hospital in Oregon, which is unfamiliar to her. She's lost a lot of confidence in the local doctors after this last incident.

Some of the doctors in California are inclined for us to stay at Children's Hospital for her bone marrow test. But I'd like to go home for a while. I know the medical team has to assess her visually every so often to know what's going on, but she's here now, OK, look at her. I don't want to have to come back to Children's Hospital in two weeks. Everything is up in the air right now. I hope we turn into one of the families who gets by without lots of complications.

For me, I probably avoid thinking too much about how I really feel about Jenny having cancer. I think I am afraid that my feelings would be debilitating to me if I were to give them full reign. Especially in hospitals, dealing with the medical professionals, I'm the one who must be in control. I'm the one who needs to reason and make decisions. It's important to me that the doctors respect me and my judgment. I always have the sense that the hospital staff is assessing me, especially the staff psychologist or the social worker. I'm conscious of how I behave around them. I'm afraid that if I let my emotions out, then I won't be as controlled as I need to be. I know I need to acknowledge that this *is* affecting me emotionally, but I still feel like I need to be in control.

One evening after Jenny received chemotherapy, she had a dozen serious seizures. No one knew why she was having them. It wasn't expected. It wasn't part of the program that was laid out to me. Her condition deteriorated rapidly. We didn't know if epilepsy had developed, or if it was a drug reaction, or if it indicated central nervous system relapse. It was several days before she was coherent and responsive. While Jenny was in the hospital recuperating from the seizures, several infections took hold. She had sores in her mouth that became so bad she couldn't swallow or eat. We had to have her transported by air ambulance to the hospital in California. At that point, I knew that these infections could kill Jenny. Most kids who died while in the middle of chemotherapy usually die from infections. I don't think that Jenny knew that. It really scared me.

Then, when her MRI scan came back abnormal, it really sent me over the edge. I thought, "That's it. There is an infection in her brain or it's a stroke." I didn't feel capable of dealing with the bad news by myself. That was when I realized that death was a possibility. I had always believed that there would be some sort of orderly progression to death, but I wasn't ready for the seizures and the infections. I knew that an infection in the brain could cause blindness, and I saw all of the horrible possibilities, and suddenly, all of those possibilities became real. I felt knocked off balance, afraid of losing control. I felt that if someone came in with one more piece of bad news, I wouldn't be able to bear it. I called Greg at home and told him that I needed his support. He came down that night.

Jenny really wasn't aware or together enough to know what was going on. We were pretty straight with Jenny about everything, but I didn't think there was much to be gained by telling her that things could really get worse. There was that added burden of trying to appear as calm and normal as possible with her. Meanwhile, other people in the family were calling and saying, "Oh, I hear Jenny's condition is really bad."

Then, when I got home after Jenny was discharged from the hospital, I felt like I always had to be on guard for another emergency. I wasn't going to let myself be surprised the next time. I was determined to be

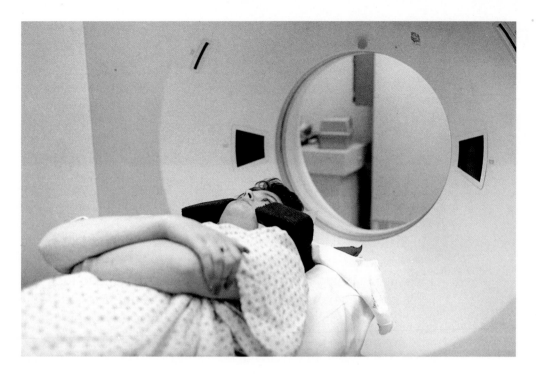

Jenny gets a CAT scan to check the progress of her cancer treatment.

ready for anything. I was trying to have a normal life, but inside I was always on the alert. All of this exhausted me, and I was so tired I could barely function. I felt like I was walking on an icy lake. Then I realized that I couldn't hold myself ready at all times, but I know I'm more ready than I ever was.

Not being committed outside the family helps me to feel less pressured. Jenny's illness has been my reason for backing out of things I was involved in. For the most part, that feels like a relief, although sometimes I feel that urge to get involved again. It's hard because I know that Jenny is looking at this and thinking, "I'm causing this. My mom's not involved in theater because of my illness. I'm disrupting the family." I try to be honest with her and reassure her that this is just life. It's not her fault. There is no guilt and no blame. I can't pretend the illness doesn't disrupt us or that the bills aren't a problem. Jenny is almost an adult, and she's aware of it. All I can do is say, "Hey, no problem. I don't mind not being involved in things right now. You're more important."

My perception is that Jenny may compare herself to other teenagers who are sick. Of the two people she knew best in the hospital, one has died and the other quite possibly has also died. The first girl's death

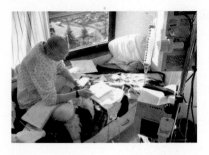

Due to chemotherapy complications, Jenny has an extended hospital stay in isolation.

was a blow to Jenny. They had a lot in common. They shared a room, and a disease. It was pretty horrible.

I know that Jenny needs the independence of any 17-year-old teenager. At the same time, there are always fearful thoughts in the back of my head that something could happen and we should always be around. I feel a tremendous amount of pressure. People tell me that being on the maintenance chemotherapy schedule is much easier. I've cautiously believed that.

Now, Jenny is on a maintenance schedule. That means she needs to see a doctor every twenty-eight days for a push of vincristine. And she takes methotrexate, prednisone, and 6-MP at home. We're actually going in the hospital less often than before. We see the doctor in town, and he is perfectly capable of doing everything, and he doesn't charge as much. We are learning how Jenny's body is responding to these chemicals. For instance, ten days after her vincristine she tends to feel really bad.

Through all of this, I think it has probably been the most difficult for our son, Jeremy. In day-to-day life he gets the brunt of responsibilities and chores that Jenny is not doing. I try to be as fair as possible, but there is a fine line. Jenny does not have much energy. On the other hand, if she can socialize and do other things, then she has the energy to help. Jeremy just has to deal with the fact that sometimes he's got to do more work. There is some resentment, but he knows he can't blame it on Jenny.

Jeremy and Rebekah just came back from an oncology siblings camp. I think Jeremy's looking at Jenny's illness differently now. Before, he avoided considering the possibility that she might die. For the two girls, I think the hardest thing to deal with was the separation when Jenny was first in the hospital. They are afraid that something will take us away again.

Each of us feels the pressure differently. The financial burden lies heaviest on Greg, and the girls worry about us being gone. I think that Jeremy probably feels the most isolated. The girls are able to get comfort from us in a way that Jeremy can't, or won't, ask for. He's been very open with us about what went on at camp. He said it's absolutely changed the way he looks at cancer.

Sometimes it seems like Jenny would rather not deal with the issue of being sick. I'm the one who reads and recommends the books. I don't know if she isn't interested, or if she feels like I'll get all the information.

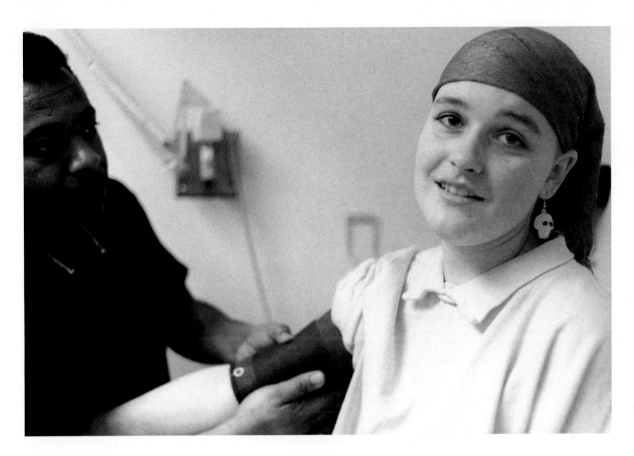

Jenny's hospital nurse takes her blood pressure.

This year, when she was feeling really bad, we wanted to reduce her school schedule to half a day. She absolutely refused to do it and really made a stink. I wonder if that is because she is reluctant to acknowledge the impact cancer has had on her life. But it's important that she realize that she is sick, that she has a Broviac—a vein implant—and that she has to take her medicine.

 Jenny doesn't take care of her mouth as well as she is supposed to in order to prevent sores. I guess she thinks, "I hate to stop and think that I have to do this because I've got cancer." Meanwhile, I'm asking, "Do you know what an infection in your Broviac tubes means? Do you need me to flush it for you every day, or do I just have the doctors take it out?" That is an option for her, but she doesn't want it taken out. She wants to avoid getting a shot. I think Jenny focuses her pain and anxiety on the small details. She'll have fits over having her finger poked for a blood test when she's been through much more horrible procedures. Maybe that's

27

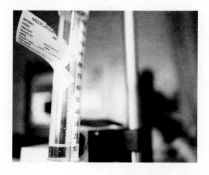

just where she can let out that anxiety or complain. It's hard to just let her be that person and do those things. We are so enmeshed, it's difficult to separate from each other.

I feel like a better parent now. There was a time when I felt more in control of my children's lives. I'm less inclined to do that now. Before, it was more important to me that everyone go along with the program and behave. I would give up being their friend for obedience. Now, I choose to be the friend. Some of the things Jenny did before, like go out with a guy, or go to the mall with a friend, have lost their importance. This thing now is so much larger.

I'm concerned that this illness has absorbed me to the point where I don't have much left for the other children, especially the girls. I hope they weather it and use this experience for the good. It could go either way, but it's out of my control. Through all of this I have always believed in God's purpose, although I don't look for a "lesson." I still feel like life is divinely ordered, and I see the possibility for personal growth. Jenny can learn to look at the bright side in the midst of her own dilemma. My other kids can learn about being selfless.

I resent the fact that this seems like it's never going to end. But I feel like the good is going to outweigh the bad. I hope I'm not being overly optimistic. But you do get a sense of the transient nature of life and relationships, and you are more inclined to take advantage of right now, to appreciate and live for the moment. I try to stop and look at all the little blessings daily, and I allow them to touch me. I also appreciate what people are doing on our behalf. I'm saying all this with the belief that we've seen the worst of it and at the end of two years it will be over. Then I can sigh with relief.

July 1991

Nine months after Jenny's diagnosis, I visit her in Klamath Falls, Oregon, and go camping with her and her family. We camp near a beautiful lake and we have a great time swimming, playing, and just relaxing as a family. Jenny is feeling better and is happy to be on a camping trip, away from the daily routine. At the end of the weekend, Jenny and I sit down at the kitchen table, alone, and she updates me on how she is doing.

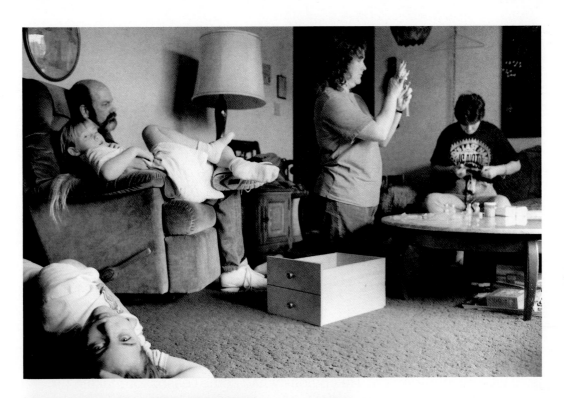

Jenny and her mother prepare the chemotherapy injection in the living room while family members watch. Then Jenny injects herself with chemotherapy drugs. Needles are discarded into a special plastic container.

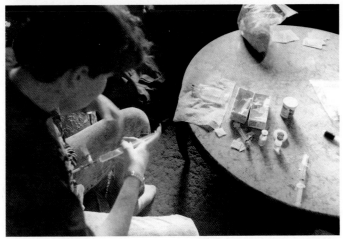

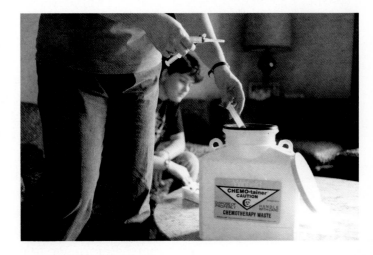

Jenny

The last time I was in the hospital with seizures and mouth sores, it showed me how quickly everything can change. I don't remember much of what happened. I only found out later how serious it was. One nurse told me she didn't think I was going to make it. But at the time it was happening, I didn't think of that.

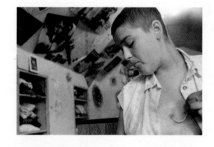

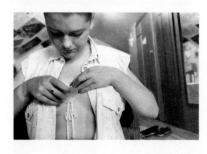

I'm not afraid of dying. I think it would be cool to, like, die, and then see who comes to my funeral. I don't think about it much. I don't fear it. Just because I have cancer doesn't mean I have to die. Each case is different, and each person isn't doomed. Everyone is an individual. If you make it or not, it's what's supposed to happen. Everyone is going to die, you can't change that. The doctors tell me I've got a 30 percent chance of not making it. So what? That doesn't mean anything to me. I don't dwell on it.

My faith in God helps me a lot. I don't know how people do this without God. Little miracles happen when I pray. Sometimes I feel down, I get tired of staring at the wall, watching TV. Sometimes I ask Him for just a little encouragement. He obviously had some reason for making me sick. Maybe it was to change my life, or my family's life, or someone else's life. You can get a lot out of illness. You find out what you are capable of, how strong you really are, who your friends are. I don't feel like I've been stopped from anything.

People tell me I've got such a great attitude. They don't see me when I complain. There are times when I don't feel so well, but I try not to show it to everybody. Everyone tells me I've got mood swings. They say it's from the chemo. Maybe it is, but I keep the really huge mood swings to myself. I don't let anyone know about those. When I was in the hospital, I felt like I could show my moods. I could say what hurt and what was OK. But when I'm out, I don't want to say anything because I don't want to go to the doctor again. I know the price of drugs, I know how expensive everything is. I didn't want my dad to get stuck with all these bills. I just have to keep reminding myself that I really need these things and they'll get paid for somehow.

I feel kind of responsible that my brother, Jeremy, gets the brunt of everything now, especially chores around the house. He's trying so hard. Before, we teamed up. But now he's doing it alone. When I had the seizures, Jeremy helped a lot. I think he is very scared of losing me. He's just beginning to realize the weight of the situation.

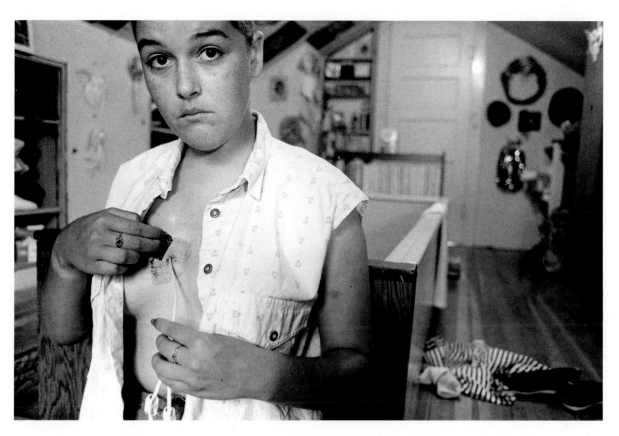

Jenny cleans her
Broviac vein
implant, a part of
her daily routine.

     I try not to use the disease as a crutch to get out of things, but I am a lot lazier now. Like school. I'm going to go ahead and take an extra year of high school. I'll be a senior this year, and again next year. I won't be graduating with my class, which is kind of a bummer. I wasn't there much during my junior year. I don't use the cancer to get out of courses, but if I even feel the least bit tired, I blow them off. Then I feel guilty when I go out with friends or something. I have to work really hard to do my homework, to finish the things I start, while trying to enjoy life, too.

     As far as I'm concerned, I don't think anyone deserves to be sick. I just want to make sure that people don't say or do things for me just because of that. I don't want anything out of pity. I don't like how, now, everybody's nice to me, especially at school. I don't feel like I'm better than anyone else or that I deserve more sympathy. I want people to tell it like it is, just like I would do for them. I expect that from everyone, especially my doctors. There are a lot of people out there who are a lot worse off than me. I don't know why I'm looked at as the recipient of the worst thing in the world.

31

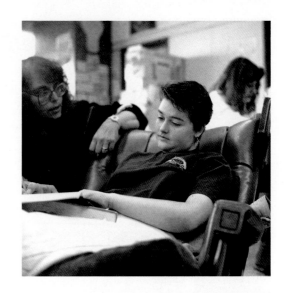

Jenny at school with
her teacher.

This disease has made me really insecure about myself. I always have to make sure I clearly understand what the other person is saying or meaning. I'm afraid I might interpret something wrong. I'm always saying I'm sorry. I feel like I'm complaining when someone asks me how I'm doing. I don't want to feel sorry for myself. And I'm so self-conscious now. I hate being fat. It drives me crazy. The prednisone makes me eat a lot. And when I got sick I couldn't dance or do anything physical. I lie in bed a lot now. I can see my body changing. My stomach is not as flat. My waist is not as thin as it was. My legs are like watermelons! I know some of it is because I'm getting older, but if I wasn't sick, I'd be running around as much as always.

Being bald doesn't bother me. When I first lost my hair, I wore scarves. Now I wear baseball caps all the time. I never wear a wig. And now that I'm on maintenance, my hair is coming in again. Everyone thinks it's so hip to have such short hair. I joke around about it. I asked a barber for a trim when we were in the Bahamas, but he didn't think it was funny. It's growing in now, but it could fall out at any time.

I've been on maintenance now for two months, and it's still growing. On maintenance, I'm taking a lot of the same drugs as I was in the beginning. I still get vincristine, prednisone, IV methotrexate, oral methotrexate, 6-MP. Most of them are in pill form, some in IV, some are given in spinal taps. Every three months I get a spinal with IV methotrexate. I'll still be getting bone marrows once in a while. This is only my second month

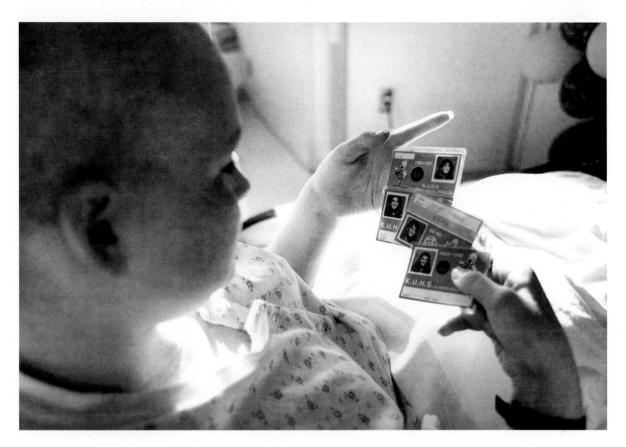

Jenny looks at
high school ID
photos of herself
and recalls how
she looked
before her
cancer.

on this schedule, so I don't know how this will change. Now I get more
drugs, but maybe not such a high dose, or as often. Now my side effects
aren't as extreme.

Compared to the beginning of my treatment, this is a breeze. For
the first six months the side effects were horrible. Really intense. First I
gained a lot of weight; I was really gassy from the drugs; I had joint pain;
my muscles would cramp. I had a lot of mucus buildup, and it hurt my
stomach and throat.

Now my weight varies a lot. I still take prednisone, and it makes
me eat and eat, so I go up and down when I'm on and off that. Sometimes
I feel nauseated. It makes me not want to do anything. The sun and the
heat bother me, they give me headaches. But it's a lot nicer to be out of
the hospital and be able to socialize. I'm able to do things and go out
when I feel good. One of my favorite things is to go on patrol with the
Coast Guard. When I feel good, I can also go to school. I used to be on

the swim team, but because of my Broviac, and not being as strong as I used to be, I'm not doing that this summer.

I still can't try out for theater. I never know if in the middle of it I'll get sick and have to leave. There are a lot of things I'd love to be involved in now but can't. I don't know if I'll ever be able to get back into my interests in high school. Once I'm in college I won't have the same schedule. I feel like I'm missing out on stuff that I won't be able to pick up on for a long time. You have to have a sense of humor to get through these things. A lot of people can't laugh, especially about having no hair. You've just got to say, "Hey, this is the way it is." I think having my mom, who is so positive, helps a lot. I think it's important to live for the moment. There are so many people who schedule everything, a routine they never break. You have to seize the moment but also find a balance.

People ask me what is the worst thing about having cancer. I don't know. *What is the worst thing about living your life?* You have to live your life with cancer the way you would without it. You need to pay attention to your limitations while trying to live as normally as possible. Use the illness to its advantage. There are a lot of pros. Sure, I'd rather not have it, but since I do, I have to make the best of it. You meet other people who have it. You get to know the people who recognize the important things in life. You can talk to doctors and nurses and increase your knowledge. You can gain insight into what other people might be going through. Your family might become closer. You can do some public speaking about your illness. There are a lot of good things that can come from being sick. I know there are people who only think about dying. "Poor me," they say all the time. Give it up. Get off it.

July 1991

After returning from the weekend camping trip, I pull Jenny's dad, Greg, aside and ask to speak with him alone. We find a quiet spot in the comfortable family room in the basement of their home. I want to hear how it has been for him as Jenny's father, watching his daughter go through cancer treatments. Greg is candid and friendly, willing to talk about himself and his feelings.

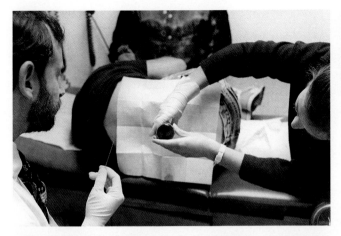

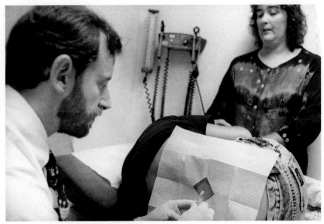

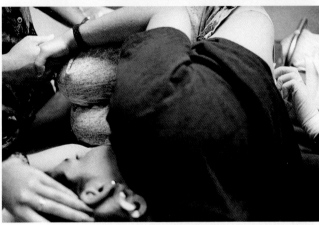

The doctor prepares Jenny for a spinal tap (top left). He taps the spine for fluid by using a long needle. Jenny's family offers support during the spinal tap because it can be a painful procedure.

Greg, Jenny's father

When Jenny was first diagnosed with cancer I lived in shock. In the very beginning I was willing to throw out everything in my life because nothing else really mattered. The health of my kid is primary. I just walked away from work and let somebody else finish what I was doing. Fortunately, while I was getting through the first part of this shock, I got to hide away in isolation for a bit in the hospital. It's a real helpless feeling. I wanted to be able to protect my kid and hold her and comfort her. I felt helpless. There is nothing I can do except be an emotional support.

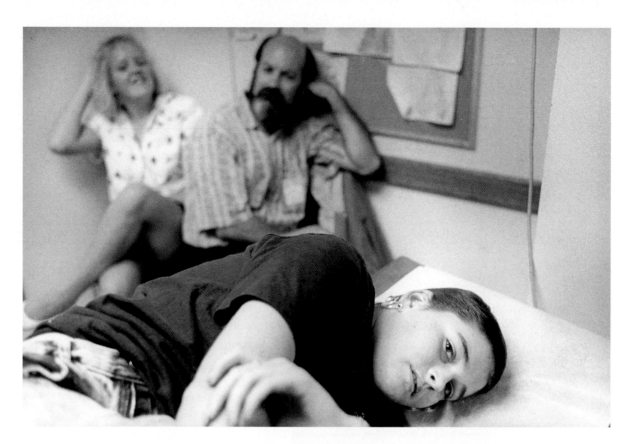

Jenny rests after the spinal tap with a friend and her father, Greg.

In the beginning we did stand by the bed and hold Jenny and brush her forehead when she was in pain. But I still felt helpless. Then I got to the point when I realized that I had to go out of the hospital. That's kind of a scary feeling, to go back out into a world where everything is going on just like the day before Jenny was diagnosed, but nothing is really the same. It's very scary.

I really had to put my head down and force myself to get back into my daily schedule. Nothing comes naturally at first. There is a helpless feeling of, What difference does it make? Why even bother? Why should I go to work because no matter how much I work I can't pay the bills anyway? It's like playing fifty-two-card pick-up with your life. Everything is thrown up into the air, and everything is irrelevant. Nothing matters, but you still have to go on.

When Vicki was down in California at the hospital, I was home calling friends. Calling and telling people is a real struggle. It's really hard to call a friend and when they ask what's new, tell them my daughter has cancer. I never know how they are going to react. The friends who broke into tears were the ones who really got to me. Immediately the pain was being shared. It really chokes me up when they are right there with me, suffering, carrying that load, asking what they can do.

I never know when my emotions are going to overcome me. I can be having a conversation and suddenly a word, a thought, something comes up where I'm just blinded by my emotions. I've got a lump in my throat, I can't talk, tears are rolling down my cheeks. It's different from week to week, day to day. That was hard at the very beginning because I was afraid to talk about it, afraid of the feelings, but I wanted to talk about it with people I'm close to.

The first couple of months into the disease were real emotional. I dealt with it emotionally, not medically, like Vicki tends to do. I was home with the kids, I was getting and giving the calls, telling people what was going on. It's really humbling to be able to let yourself cry on the phone, in person, to talk to somebody, and just cry. It's a great release.

It's too bad more men can't cry. I've had conversations with Jenny where in the middle of it I've got tears rolling down my cheeks. One time I said, "You know, I don't know what you expect from me. I don't know if you want me to have this big macho image where you look at me and want me to have everything in control. I feel helpless. I want to be able to help you, to comfort you, to do all these things. I hurt like you can't believe, and I would rather let you see me cry, see there are emotions there. I don't mind you seeing me when I feel sensitive and vulnerable. I don't want to hide it from you." At times it seems like it would be easier to be the one who has cancer. You don't worry the same way.

Sometimes I see incredible competence and compassion around Jenny, and that's a great thing. But sometimes I see bumbling stooges. Often I have to leave the room. I try to do a good job in my trade by keeping up on the latest techniques in order to constantly improve myself, and when I don't see that in the medical profession, I lose patience. They are dealing with people's lives, I am dealing with people's houses. At times I see people taking less care with my daughter's life than I take with someone's house. That's real hard for me. But at other times, I see wonderful things. I walked in on a nurse who was making Jenny's bed and there was a tear rolling down her cheek. When I see Jenny's nurse crying from emotion, that's a grabber.

37

If I could say something to other parents, it would be to let your emotions out. What do you have to lose, anyway? If your friends are awkward because you're letting your tears out and they can't handle it, then they're not your friends anyway. Your kid is better off seeing you cry, better off seeing you call a friend and say, "I just need somebody to sit with me and talk." They're better off knowing that you have ups and downs because they do, too.

You do get past that emotional mountain. And it does start to mellow out a little bit. But you always have this dark cloud hanging over you. I know that God doesn't heal every kid, and that's really frustrating. You can pray for your kid all the time. We talk to other people on the oncology floor, and they've told us how many times their kids have been back in the hospital and what they were in for. So yes, we know what can happen. Jenny wakes up one morning and she feels halfway decent, and suddenly one day she doesn't. I think, "My God, we could lose her right now." I don't dwell on her dying every day, but I know it's a possibility. It never really leaves.

We focus more on doing things. We are spur-of-the-moment people. Even more so now. We grab those little chunks of time when Jenny's got a good attitude and is feeling OK—those good moments come between chemotherapy treatments—and make the best of them. Sure, it's not fair to our other kids. If it was fair, Jenny wouldn't have cancer. Yes, sometimes someone else in our family gets excluded, but there is no way to have your other kids understand that it's better to have nothing and not have cancer than to have cancer and get tons of gifts. I can explain it all you want, but I am talking to children who see treats and gifts.

It's frustrating when I don't really have time to do all the things I want to do with all our kids. It's a no-win situation. You'd better hope as a parent that you've said "I love you" to your kids enough times before a crisis happens. When they're laying there in the hospital, it's too late if you haven't said it and given them all your hugs before. It's like a savings account. Don't put off little things. Maybe nothing will ever happen, but if it does, you're going to kick yourself for a long time.

Even now, we spend money on stuff that we shouldn't spend it on. Who knows if Jenny is going to live five years, ten years, two weeks? We see changes in her, mood swings. Real mood swings—not just up-and-down days. It happens on a large scale. We'll be talking, joking, and suddenly she stomps out of the room, mad at everybody. Also, in the middle of a conversation Jenny blanks out. She drifts in and out of the topic, and we don't know where she is. We don't know if it's permanent and if it is, so what? I try not to focus on that stuff, but who knows if she's sterile or if her kids will have birth defects? I have to force myself not to worry about those things. Instead, I tell myself, today, right now, she's feeling good, she's alive. What can we do today?

I want other parents to know that this is an emotional struggle. If you allow yourself to become vulnerable and show your feelings at the start, it makes dealing with it later much easier. You have to let people see you as vulnerable. If you build a wall, if you hide from your friends, if you keep your emotions inside, six months later the wall just gets bigger and you become more irritated with people for not calling, not doing things, not reacting, whatever.

People don't know what to do. It was amazing for me to realize how few friends I really have. I mean real friends. People who will drop everything and drive an hour, three hours, whatever. They'll ask, "Hey, do you need any money?" And they'll send a check. You don't have a lot of those people in your life. There are a lot of people who say they want to help, but don't. I don't say anything to people like that, but I want to say, "Send a dinner over. Vicki's gone and I work all day. I get home at seven-thirty after picking up kids all around town and doing errands. I don't want to cook dinner, and it would be nice if you could drop off dinner."

It was nice to see people mail cards to Jenny directly, without me having to say something. It cheered her up. It's nice to see people doing things like that. Sometimes people are incredibly rude and thoughtless. It's so irritating to see what people do and say to Jenny when she has no hair, when she is out in public with nothing on her head. Jenny has got guts. Sometimes you just want to be a bodyguard. Sometimes I want to yell at people because they're so offensive. I can't do that, and I can't always protect my child.

I would hope all pediatric floors are as good as the one at Children's Hospital in Oakland. I've met some really great people—nurses and doctors who give us a lot of help. In the hospital, some people want to hide, and some people don't, they want to talk. We have been lucky to meet good, helpful people. Now that we've gone through it with Jenny,

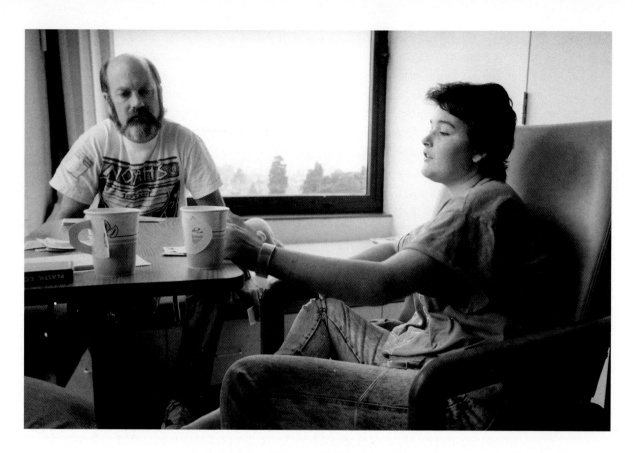

Greg with
his daughter
Jenny.

we want to help others if we can. If someone came to us whose kid had cancer, we'd be able to explain some things to them. We've been through the first six months now, and we feel like veterans of the cancer ward.

Sometimes it surprises Jenny when I refer to this whole experience as "we." The whole family is included. It's different for us, but our lives are affected, also. Nothing will ever be the same. I try to feel like I've got a normal family. On the other hand, I know I don't. But life goes on. Emotionally, the parents can die and never come out of it, just like the child can die physically. It's a shame that people let themselves die emotionally when something like this happens.

Vicki and I connect with Jenny on different levels. There are times when we're both trying to boost her up from different directions. One of us can usually always talk to Jenny, but sometimes she doesn't want either of us around, so I try to be sensitive to what she needs. Fortunately, we've never all been down at the same time.

Before Jenny was diagnosed with cancer she was a normal teen. She didn't want to be seen with her mom or dad. She didn't want to talk to us. Now Jenny realizes she needs the emotional support from us. We don't hide the medical bills from her. Jenny is old enough to pick up the bills and see what things cost. I don't mind if she sees them, but I don't want her to dwell on them. We try never to complain about the medical costs, not only because we don't want her to see us complain, but because it's a destructive path and it's not going to help. Sure, it feels like we're going to be in the poorhouse forever. But we're not living in our car. We still have a house to live in. We have grocery money.

For me, there is no explanation for sickness and death and dying. I know there is a God, and I can accept certain things. I try not to ask, "God, why haven't you healed my kid?" Maybe he's going to allow the chemo to heal her—I don't know. It's certainly a test of faith. You have to plow through a lot of things in life, and hopefully you can plow through with God. I have to remind myself to be grateful for small things. It can't be all or nothing. One day Jenny and Vicki were waiting to go to the hospital, and this old man turned around and gave Vicki twenty dollars. We didn't know him. He allowed himself to go with his gut feeling, which too many people bury for fear of being embarrassed. When people do go with their gut emotion, it really chokes me up. When someone does send a card or a five-dollar bill it means so much to me. You've got to be able to keep your eyes open to the small stuff because the small victories are more frequent with chemo. If you can't see that, you're going to be a mess.

Some parts of my life changed a lot, and some parts didn't. In the end, I hope Jenny would see that I'm willing to drop work and do what it takes. She's not a verbal person. She can't say, "I love you." At times she's hard to figure out. We get along a lot better than before. We talk a lot more now. I think a lot of that is the result of taking time off from work and just standing next to her in the hospital. It's hard to watch your kid curl up having convulsions, or become comatose from chemo.

Cancer is devastating to marriages. There is a horrible percentage of families who don't stay together. Everything is magnified. It's important that things are good in the relationship before the illness. Under the pressure of dealing with cancer, things can get explosive. I really believe that if you don't have a good relationship beforehand you're not going to get it when things get rough.

My relationship with my wife, Vicki, has changed in some ways. The changes are scary and comforting at the same time. I never know what's going to happen in our marriage because everything outside of it is so exaggerated. Sure, I can say we've got a good marriage, and we'll never split up, but I don't know that. I never know what's going to trigger a change, for better or worse. I try to hang on to it while it's there and do everything I can. It's the same as trying to stock up all your hugs and love on your kid before the illness so that when a crisis hits, you make it through.

The main thing is if you persevere in your day-to-day life and in your relationships, things do get better. Life doesn't get normal again the way it was before, but we're back to doing normal things when Jenny's feeling well. It's a scary thing when Jenny has been in the hospital and a few weeks later she wants to get up and start doing things. I know how vulnerable she is, and I want to protect her, but I know she has to get out and do things, see her friends. I think the biggest thing parents can do for their kids is offer encouragement for them to be with their friends. To hang on to a little bit of the old life that was normal before cancer.

In the very beginning, when Jenny was losing her hair from chemo, she wore a scarf. It was awkward knowing she didn't have any hair and knowing she was getting the looks. I think parents can be too much of an influence on what their kid does when they lose their hair, telling them to wear a hat, get a wig, cover it up. The first time I took Jenny to the mall without a wig it felt weird, and out of the corner of my eye, I could see heads spinning. I realize Jenny's got to decide for herself when she should cover her head. I don't know why it seems easier for her than for other kids. If somebody said ten months ago that Jenny would walk around in public with no hair. . . . Before she got cancer she spent so long in front of the mirror every morning we'd have to bang down the door. How can you ever guess anything like this could ever happen? Yes, her hair will grow long again. Jenny is really pretty, and she's got a face that can go in public without any hair. And she's doing it.

For other parents going through this, my advice is to force yourselves to verbalize your emotions with a few friends. Yeah, it does feel pretty lopsided when you're in need and you're the one making the phone calls. But most of the time, you are the one who has to call out. Hopefully you can do it. Struggle through the anger as fast as you can.

Pray. Accept it. It's there. You're not going to change it. Hopefully you can find doctors you're comfortable with. That's a big part of it. Talk to them. Ask questions. Find out what's going on and what's going to happen. Don't be surprised by what can happen. Look into the books and learn about the disease. Don't let the lump in your throat or the tears in your eyes prevent you from talking to people. And remember that life goes on. Take every day and make the best of it.

July 1991

At one point on the camping trip, I sit down with Jenny's younger sisters, both bright and articulate, and talk with them about Jenny's cancer and how it affects them.

Joanna, Jenny's sister, age 8
Rebekah, Jenny's sister, age 10

How did you feel when you heard your sister had leukemia?

Joanna: It was scary. I didn't know what was going to happen to her.

Rebekah: I didn't know what leukemia was.

Joanna: We asked Dad about it. We asked what it was. I didn't know that it is a type of cancer.

Rebekah: I didn't even know how to say leukemia because I'd never heard of it before. We talked to Dad because he was the only one at home.

Joanna: I came home from soccer practice one day and found out that Mom and Jenny were gone. They were away at the hospital for three months. We wanted them to come back. We talked to them almost every day. It was really weird to see Jenny with no hair. I'd never seen anyone like that before.

Rebekah: I'd never seen anyone bald except for Dad, and he's not even totally bald. I've also noticed that Jenny's kind of white. She used to have a good tan, and now she's white.

What else have you noticed about Jenny that has changed?

Joanna: Well, I think she's getting along with Mom and Dad better.

Rebekah: I think she's getting along with them better, but not with us. I don't know why.

Joanna: I think it's because they've had to spend a lot of time together lately. I wish I would get the presents Jenny gets sometimes. I do feel left out once in a while.

Rebekah: One thing though, we always have to do whatever Jenny wants to do. If she wants to lay on the bed that we're on, then we have to get off.

Joanna: When we went to visit her in the California hospital it was nice because we were getting along better there. Her personality hadn't seemed to change so much. But now, at home, it's back to normal with us.

Rebekah: It seems strange to see her bald and then to see her with hair. We are getting used to seeing her Broviac and having to clean and dress it every day.

Joanna: I think it's neat to watch that. We've learned a lot from Jenny being sick. I've learned about the disease. I hadn't ever heard of it before this.

How do you think it's affected you personally?

Rebekah: Things are different. A lot different. Everything's changed like I never thought it would. Like, I never thought Jenny would lose her hair.

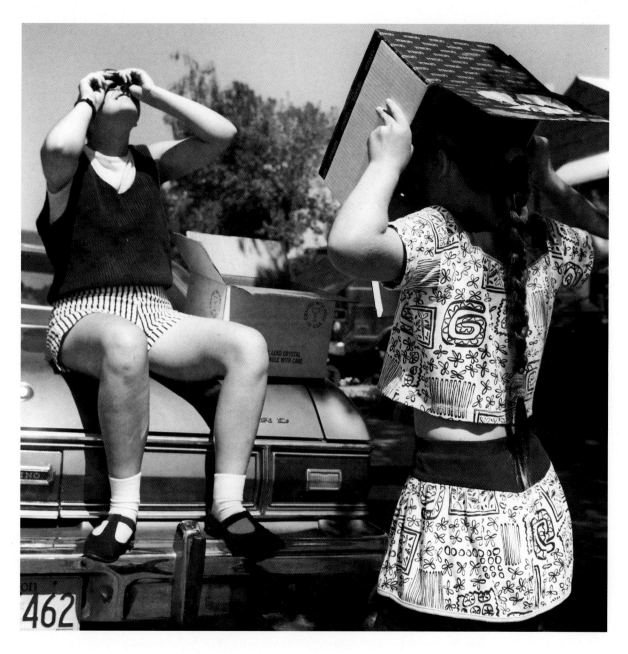

Jenny and her
sister Joanna
watch an eclipse
of the sun while
protecting their
eyes from direct
exposure.

45

Joanna: I feel like I'm closer to my mom and dad now. I talk to them more, ask them lots of questions. Usually it's about sickness and what Jenny's going through.

Rebekah: I wish it never happened to my family.

Joanna: I don't know. It's hard to say that. I've gained something. I think sometimes it would be better if she never got sick, and sometimes I think it's good she did get sick. I think it's gotten our family closer. We're all growing closer to Mom and Dad and Jenny, so it's good. One time I took a card for Jenny to school and everybody signed it.

Rebekah: Jenny came to my class once. She just sat there, and everybody asked her questions. Some of the kids in the other classes stood at the door and watched.

Joanna: I think it's good that she doesn't cover her hair up.

Rebekah: Yeah, she took her hat off in my classroom, and she takes it off in public. No one laughs. Some of the kids she used to baby-sit for don't even recognize her anymore. They are scared of her. They'd never seen her bald. Jenny said the drugs that get rid of the cancer are worse than the cancer itself. You can't feel the cancer, it's just there. The drugs do stuff to you. If people don't know what's wrong with Jenny, I can tell them why she lost her hair and a couple of the side effects.

Rebekah, what did you think of siblings camp?

Rebekah: There wasn't much to do except for rest hour. Once we walked down Memory Lane. There was a path cleared and some painted rocks. We walked on them. They didn't really talk to us about cancer. Camp was supposed to take our minds off that stuff. SIBS stands for Special Important Brothers and Sisters. There was this thing called "Just as Special" that each cabin did. We were supposed to come up with a sentence or poem that meant you were just as important as your sick brother or sister. I don't know what my cabin said. I wasn't paying attention.

Are you getting used to the changes you've seen in Jenny?

> **Joanna:** We think life with Jenny this way is normal now. It didn't take long. We wish she didn't have to go back into the hospital the last time when she had the seizures. It took both her and Mom away from us.

> **Rebekah:** I get used to them having to make hospital and doctor visits often. Usually Jenny goes to the doctor and gets platelet and blood transfusions and little vials of this drug called zofran. The time, two and a half years, isn't very short. That's the time that Jenny is doing something, on pills or something. Then she needs five years in remission before the doctors feel she's totally OK.

> **Joanna:** I think actually we're doing good as a family. We're growing closer together, and I think that's good. I think that's one of the best changes since Jenny's gotten sick.

July 1991

> *One afternoon during the camping trip, Jeremy and I sit on a big rock near the lake's edge, watching his family swim. Jeremy is very open to talking about his sister's cancer and how it has affected him.*

Jeremy, Jenny's brother, age 15

How do you feel about being the brother of someone with cancer?

> I feel responsible, like I have a duty. I always have to keep an eye on Jenny, just in case, for her protection from people teasing her. I've seen that before, and it really makes me upset.

Is your relationship with Jenny better now?

> Our relationship is pretty much the same because I try to keep it the same. I don't want Jenny to think I'm changing just for her. We should

treat her like a normal person. I know she needs special treatment sometimes, but she should also be treated like a normal human being.

How did you feel when you first found out Jenny was sick?

I started crying. It hit me really hard. I just didn't know what to do. It was really scary. Before then I had done a report on leukemia, so I knew a little about it. I started reading books, and now I don't feel so scared, but still a little bit.

I went to siblings camp, and most of the kids there had brothers or sisters who had died. Before I got to camp I never thought that could happen to Jenny. At least three-fourths of the kids at the camp had lost brothers or sisters. It was unreal. I felt pretty lucky. The counselors told us that our brothers and sisters could die, but they also said to take it easy and not to think about it.

What really affected me at siblings camp was how everyone was so close and we were all there for the same reasons. I liked being able to ask anyone questions and get answers. I asked, "How long will the treatments be? What are some of the side effects the doctors don't tell you about? What's it like afterwards?" Jenny's sickness has exposed me to a lot more. It's shown me that there can be nice people and that there is a lot more than what you read about in the newspapers. People have been good to my family and about talking to me. I'm definitely going back to siblings camp next year, even if she dies. I loved it. It was wonderful.

What changes have you noticed in your family since Jenny got sick?

Everyone in the family is more strained now. When Mom is gone with Jenny, everyone is on such a tight schedule. You don't really have time to do anything for yourself. I can't really ask for a ride someplace because nobody is around. I'm not really jealous. I realize it's a disease and it's life-threatening and sometimes I do feel left out, but I don't get angry.

Has your relationship with your parents changed at all?

No. It's pretty much the same. They mind their own business and so do I. My mom and I get along, but my dad—we don't get along. This sickness has really brought me and my mom closer. My sister Rebekah and I are definitely really close. It's kind of hard to explain. Jenny's illness has made me try to take everything into consideration, to look at the whole picture before you make up your mind, think about everyone and everything. I appreciate people and life a lot more. It still blows me away how many of those kids at camp lost a brother or a sister. They had this thing called Memory Lane. There were hundreds of rocks inside a pond with the names of the kids who'd died. That made me really appreciate human life.

February 1992

Jenny is in the midst of a six-week hospital stay, in isolation, because she keeps running high fevers. She also developed chicken pox and an infection in her lungs, which seriously complicate her condition. I visit her at Children's Hospital Oakland, and we talk for several hours. It is now one and a half years since Jenny was first diagnosed with cancer.

Jenny

How are you doing?

Jenny: The longer I'm here, the more hospitalish I get. I start to ache from being on the bed, just hanging around. During Christmas vacation I started having problems with my hip. A few weeks later, when I went to the pediatrician for my vincristine, I told him what was going on. He x-rayed my hip and elbow and knee. They found a spot on my tibia, which they were concerned about. They thought I had osteoporosis in my leg. I had a bone scan, which showed a hot and cold spot and what looked like a couple of fractured ribs.

We decided to come down from Oregon to California, to Children's Hospital. I had two bone marrows to make sure I hadn't relapsed. Luckily the doctor did a good job, so it didn't hurt much. They gave me a local anesthesia. I like bone marrows better than spinal taps, anyway. I can't stand the pressure from a spinal tap. Having a needle stuck in my back is no fun. Leukemia hides itself in the brain and spine, and your

49

body sets up blockers that the chemotherapy doesn't always get to. The doctors have to make sure the medicine gets into those areas. After the bone marrow, which showed that I hadn't relapsed, I started having lots of tests. Around this time I began having really high fevers of around 103.

How did you feel when the doctors talked about a relapse?

I really didn't think I had. I felt OK. I wasn't sick like I was when I was first diagnosed. I was thinking about it rationally. I was at school. I called my mom at lunch to find out the results of the bone scan. That's when she said we would have to go to Oakland. I was a little freaked out about that. I didn't want to go to California. I didn't want to leave school in the middle of the week. I went to my next class thinking, "Oh well, if I relapse, I re-lapse. It's a drag but . . ."

In the end, if I had relapsed, it would have meant a bone marrow transplant. It wasn't something I would have looked forward to, but I had a feeling that I hadn't relapsed, and I tried not to worry about it. I deal with things once they happen. I don't think about it beforehand. We were dealing with so many possibilities. Relapse was just the first word out of everyone's mouth.

I have had high fevers every night since we've gotten here. Today was the first time I've had morning fevers, too. They think that my bone deterioration is from long-term use of steroids. They won't take me off them because I need them. If in five months my body really can't take them anymore, then they'll think of taking me off them.

How does all this make you feel?

The thing with my hip really bothers me. They've said that I may lose it and have to have a fake one put in. But the fact that I need the steroids has to override the bone pain and the possibility of my bones becoming very brittle. My hip, which seems to be totally gone, bothers me. I don't want to lose it. I don't want surgery and the whole hassle. All these little things bother me. I seem to be the exception to every rule. Everything seems to hit me. I'm getting used to it, I guess.

The thing that really makes me mad is the waiting. The doctors always say that they need to wait and watch. Why can't they just get going? Why can't they do something? I need to get back to school. Some-times two days go by and I don't see a doctor. That's irritating. I can't afford to put my whole life on hold. I want to tell them that they aren't my main importance. I have other things in my life going on. I know that if I get sick I have to deal with it. If I have seizures I know everything has to wait so I can take care of that. That's just how it goes when you have a long-term disease like this. You just keep going. You continue your life until there is a complication. I accept this way of life. It won't always be like this, but that's how it is now, at least.

The doctors here are telling us that I can't see my doctor in Ore-gon anymore. They don't want anyone but the team here seeing me. Once a month I go to see the doctor in Oregon, and he pushes my che-motherapy for me. Now, the team here wants me to go to Ashland [Ore-gon], which is a couple of hours away, for the same thing. That means I miss school. Dad has to take time off from work. We have to find a baby-sitter. It will cost a fortune, not to mention how hard it will be to get over the mountain in the middle of winter. I'm a little mad at all this.

I wish I didn't have to worry about everything so much. It's all so easy. It's only a push of vincristine. Why do the doctors have to play such power games? Why does the hospital give us such trouble? I know they want us to come down here to California every month. It's just not pos-sible for us. I don't like them telling me to do everything.

Tell me how you're feeling now as opposed to a year ago.

I feel that my standards are higher towards friends, boyfriends, teachers, and people in general. This is especially true for myself. I expect more of me now—better quality of work in school, better grades. I don't pull the same crap I used to pull. I'm sure this would have eventually happened, but being sick has sped up the process. This sickness is a very maturing thing. I'm able to see situations differently than before. At the same time, I don't interact with the kids in high school like I used to. I don't feel like a high school student. I'm there, but it's not where I want to hang out or be a part of.

On the whole, it's different now than it would have been if I didn't get sick. I'd have gone on being a high school kid. I'm more for this change than against it. I don't feel like I've missed something. I think I have and can learn a lot more in this present situation. I listen to my

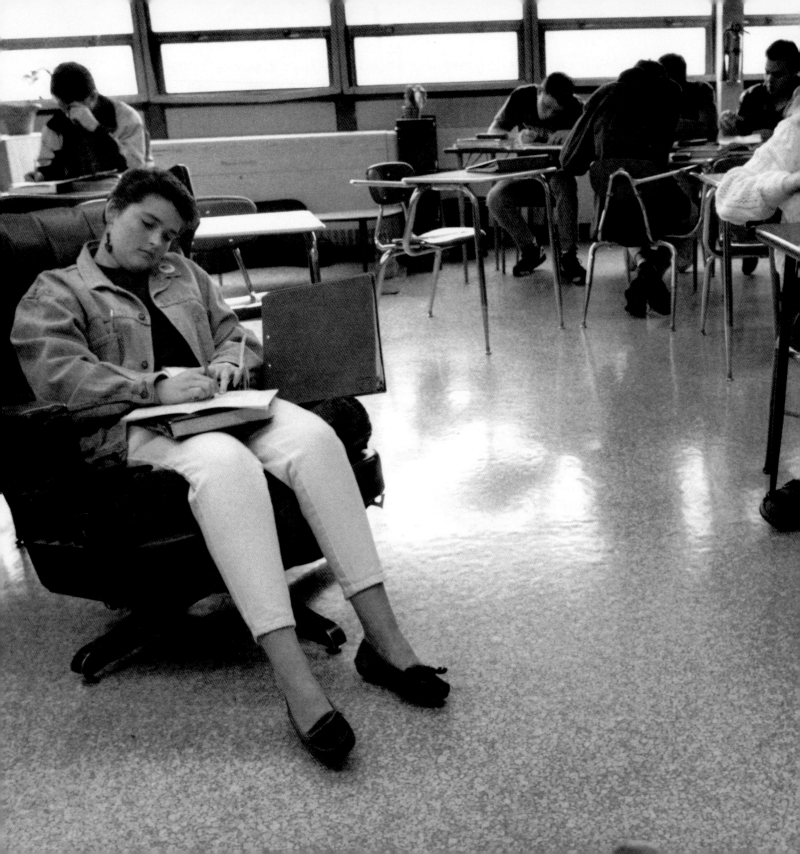

teachers. I feel a lot more intelligent now. It's my instinct to fight. I'm not worried about dying. I never thought about dying. I always fought to get past what I was going through. Right now, when I'm not really sick, I don't think about it. I don't worry. I'm more confident.

Update

Jenny was taken off chemotherapy a year earlier than scheduled because of some of the side effects of chemotherapy. The prednisone she was taking as part of her treatment protocol began to cause her bones to deteriorate. Jenny has trouble walking and will need hip and knee replacements. Despite the results, she is happy to be off chemotherapy, and feels secure about becoming well again. She spends a lot of time with her family and boyfriend and has begun taking classes at a local college. Whenever asked, Jenny continues to speak freely about her experiences with cancer.

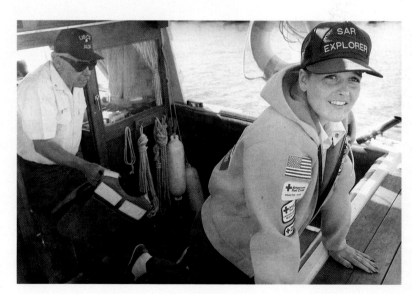

Feeling good, Jenny joins the auxiliary Coast Guard for an outing.

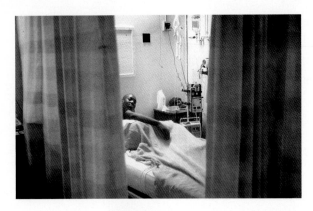

Nashawn in the
hospital during a
chemotherapy
treatment.

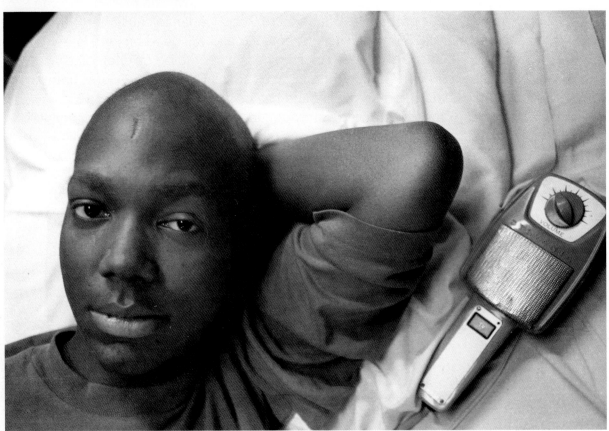

Nashawn

17 years old
Acute lymphoblastic leukemia

Nashawn is being treated for a second occurrence of leukemia at Massa-chusetts General Hospital when we first meet. He has been going through treatment for about four years, and the hospital staff claim that Nashawn is shy and quiet and probably won't speak to me about his life. But when we sit down to talk, that is not the case.

When we talk about his ordeal with cancer, Nashawn is reserved but he is certain that his experiences have made him stronger and more able to achieve his goals. We quickly learn that we share many similar experiences with cancer, and this is comforting for both of us. We get to-gether several times before I interview him, driving around Boston in my car seeing the sites or visiting with his family. I also accompany Nashawn to the hospital on several occasions when he gets his cancer treatments.

April 1989

Nashawn

What happened when you first found out you had cancer?

I was diagnosed last winter with leukemia. The name scared me. They said it was cancer. I thought I was going to die right there, I was so scared. I'd been having dizzy spells and was losing weight. I didn't know why. Then I was at McDonalds one day and fainted. I woke up and went home, but my aunt took me to the hospital where I had to stay for two weeks. I didn't speak to nobody, not even the nurses. I didn't even talk to my mom about it. It made me feel better not to talk about it. And nobody really asked me.

I don't like people to feel sorry for me. Like when the doctor would come in and joke around. He'd tell me I could get out of the hospital at a certain time, right? Then the time comes and I don't get out. I'd be mad. I hate that. I'd be telling everybody I'd be coming home, then I can't.

55

Do you talk to other teenagers who undergo chemotherapy?

No, it's boring. At home my friends ask me stupid stuff. Does it hurt? Am I going to die? A few kids died in the hospital. At first I thought that if they died, I'd die too. I don't think I'm going to, though. I just want to get cured and out of the hospital. Sometimes I wonder if I have kids, if they'll get it.

How did you feel when the cancer came back?

Terrible. I hate the hospital. I'd had treatments for one year. I was in remission. Felt back to my normal self. But then I got it back about one month ago. I had summer plans, I was going places. Now I'm tied down, all my friends are gone, nobody home to talk to. Last summer I went to Florida with a camp that's connected to the hospital. That was fun. We were at Disney World, Sea World, and Epcot Center for nine days. There were lots of kids from all over, from different hospitals. Now they've got me on this list for a bone marrow transplant. I feel yucky to think of someone else's marrow in my body. Like when I had a blood transfusion—somebody else's blood in my body. I felt strange for days. But if it cures me, I'll feel OK about it.

May 1989

Nashawn and his little brother.

During the time I spend with Nashawn, he ends up in the hospital often with fevers and infections. He also is treated with aggressive chemotherapy and ultimately, a bone marrow transplant.

A couple of weeks before Nashawn's bone marrow transplant, we sit down in the living room of his family's apartment to talk about his impending hospital stay. In addition to the unknowns of the transplant, Nashawn is also worried about his family having to move out of their house and into a housing project in a neighborhood with violence and drugs, a result of the state planning to revamp their current apartment. On top of everything else, Nashawn is worried about the safety of his younger brother and sister.

Because of the cancer treatments, Nashawn misses a lot of school, and at times he tells me he feels very left out from daily activities among his friends. However, he feels close to his large extended family, especially his mother and cousins.

56

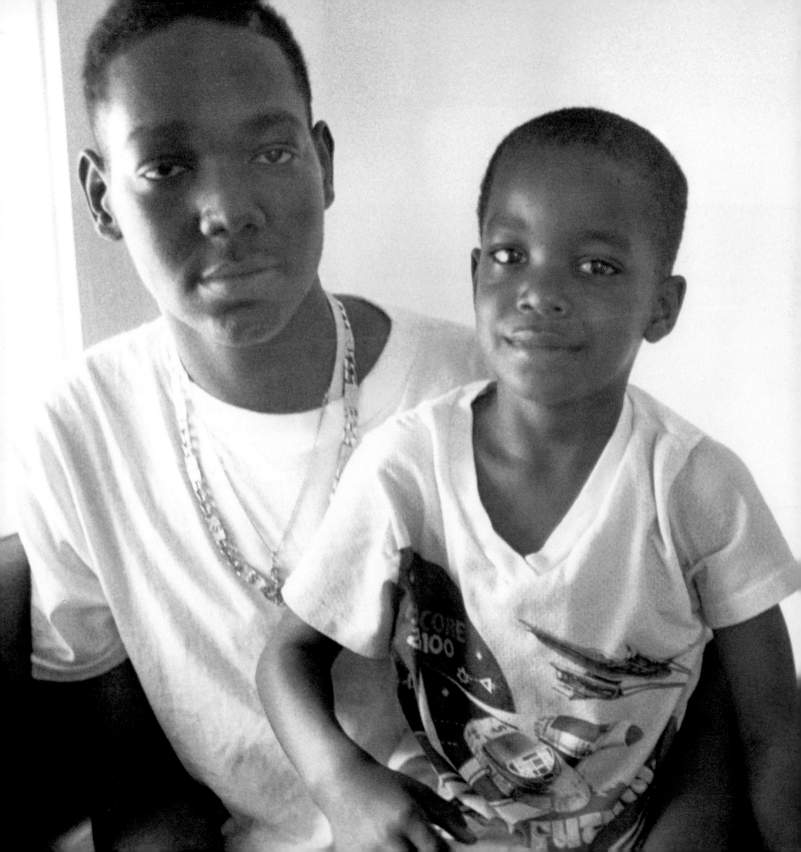

Nashawn

How do you feel about moving?

My brother and sister have grown up in our house. Me, I've lived there half my life, since we came up from the other projects. I mostly hang out with my cousins at night. They're good guys, but they're into a lot of stuff. I stay away from the stuff they're into, especially because I'm sick. I'd probably die or something. The neighborhood we have to move into is very rough. Lots of drugs. An innocent bystander can easily get hurt. Ain't nobody's fault. My mother don't want us living there, but so far she hasn't found us anything else.

When are you getting your bone marrow transplant?

Next month. They're flying me and my mother down to Maryland. I've got to stay there for about three months to see if my body accepts the transplant, and my mom has to stay with me. They won't let her come home 'cause there has to be a relative with you the whole time. I guess my aunt will take care of my brother and sister.

    I'm kind of scared, but they say my getting better is the most important thing. I guess it is. When I come back in March, my treatments will be all over. I just keep thinking of the things I'm going to do when I come home. I'll be all better then. I'll play basketball every day, be on a team I couldn't be on before, go skiing, visit lots of places I've never been. It's going to be a drag out there in Maryland, but I've just got to think of the time when I'll be out and all finished. I really think this transplant is gonna kill it, gonna knock it off for good.

September 1989

Nashawn is back from Maryland after successfully completing a bone marrow transplant. He describes the three-month hospital stay for a transplant procedure as the worst of his experiences with leukemia.

    Nashawn and his family are living in a temporary apartment while waiting for a newer one. Nashawn's mother has given him her bedroom so

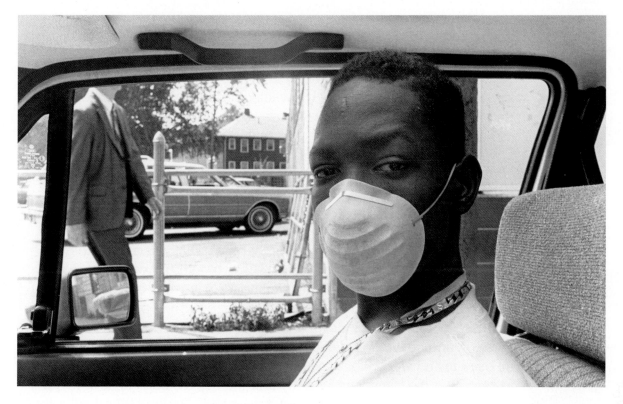

After Nashawn's bone marrow transplant, he has to wear a surgical mask while in public to protect himself against germs.

he will be more comfortable and less likely to be exposed to germs because his immune system is still recovering from the transplant. His mother sleeps with the other two children in an adjoining room. Nashawn must take a lot of medicine every day, in liquid and pill form, and a nurse visits him daily to flush his vein implant. Family members must wear surgical masks in the house, and Nashawn has to wear a surgical mask when he goes outside in order to protect himself against germs.

Nashawn

How do you feel about having to wear a surgical mask when you go somewhere?

I went to a twenty-four-hour store the other night to get something to eat. I went in wearing my surgical mask and everybody hit the ground. I walked up to the man 'cause I was in a rush. He was scared, he thought I was going to rob him or something.

59

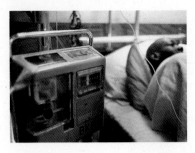

The machine in Nashawn's hospital room that regulates the flow of his chemotherapy.

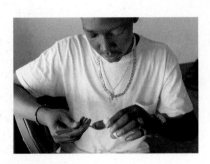

Nashawn takes an oral dose of his chemotherapy drug.

The dark ridges on Nashawn's fingernails are disappearing as his bone marrow transplant takes effect.

I haven't talked to anyone in school. They don't even know I'm home. I'd like to visit, though. This disease has messed up my last few years. It takes the fun out of life. I'm just living for the doctors, really. I've got to go to the hospital every day, and I've got to plan my day around them. I want to go to college. I'm waiting for an application to work in the park this summer. This guy wants me as his right-hand man. I've been through a lot. I mean *a lot.* I can hardly believe it. If I got through all that, I can get through anything.

Thinking back, what would you say was the worst part of your cancer treatment?

The bone marrow transplant was the hardest. That was a killer to get through. Waiting was the worst part. Three months of waiting for my blood counts to come up. All that waiting for one week of treatment. It only took a day for them to remove the marrow. They punched 200 little holes in my bones. Took out all the marrow, froze it, and treated it while I was getting heavy doses of chemotherapy for a week. Then they put it all back in and waited for it to start working. My blood counts dropped to zero after the transplant, and my hair fell out. It's back in now. It took a while, a month. That's the longest it ever took. And my blood cells are coming back. Yesterday my white blood cell count was 82,000, which means I'm getting stronger. I've got to wait till it reaches 100,000, then I won't have to wear the surgical mask anymore. And then the vein implant can come out. I'll feel like myself again.

I'm really happy my hair is back. My fingernails are better now. When the black ridges in them are gone, it means the cancer is dying. My hair feels good, nice and soft. I'm going to grow it long on top. I might get a box. That's when your hair is shaped like a box. Feels great not being tied down to the hospital. I've been going there three years and about two months.

The most painful part were the tests. Like the bladder test I had to go through. They had some gel stuff that they put on my skin, circled it around and it tells you how your bladder is moving. They were going to operate because I had so many urinary infections from the chemotherapy, but it cleared up on its own, so they didn't have to do it. The chemo is hard on your bladder and kidneys.

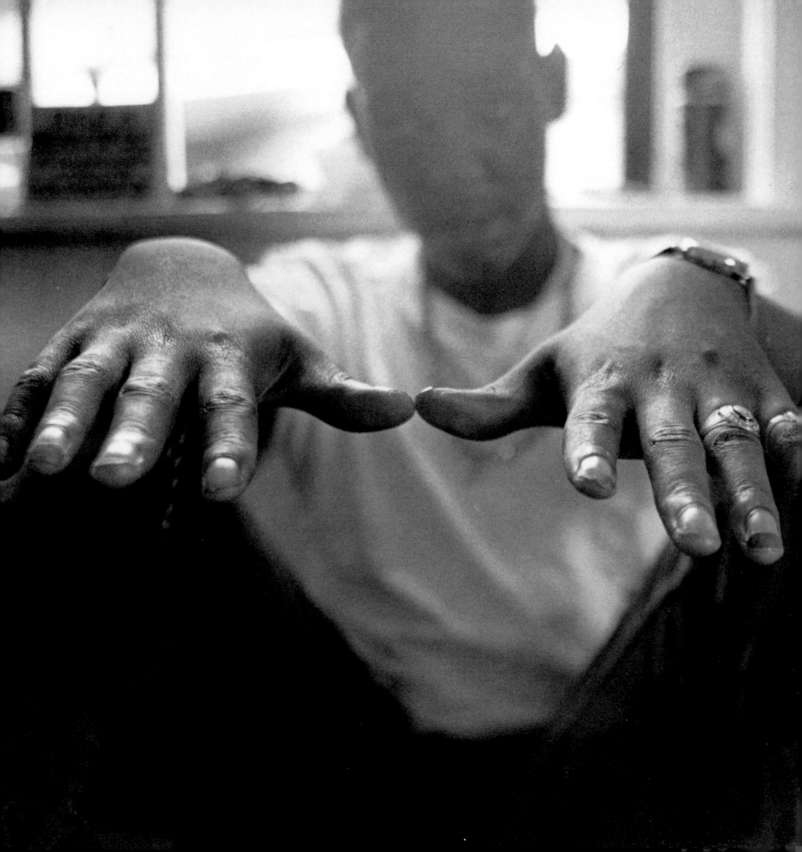

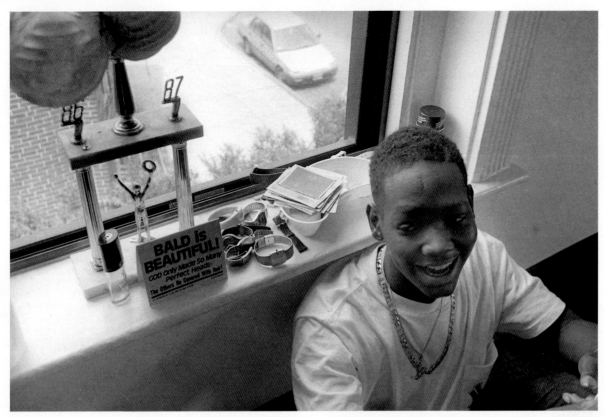

Nashawn at home.

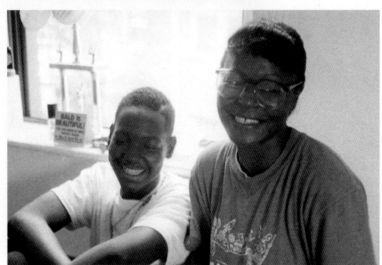

Nashawn and his mother.

Are the spinal taps painful?

Not anymore. I'm used to them now. Some days they can hurt, some days they don't. It depends on the doctor, really. They either take their time, or they have to do it over and over. The only thing I don't like is the pressure. They're digging into your marrow. I hate it when they pull back on the needle. It just pops out!

Do you have any advice for other kids who have leukemia?

Do everything the doctor tells you to do. That's how I got through. Every little detail they told me to do, I did. And don't let the depression get you down. It got to me when I was in Maryland for the bone marrow transplant. It can put you in a mood where you don't want to do nothing no more. You don't care about nothing. You just want to die. The doctors said I wasn't going to make it through. My grandmother, my mother, me, we thought I wasn't going to make it. That's a spooky feeling. I prayed a lot, that helped me. I started getting into more activities. Started riding my bike and exercising, doing my laps, talking. I kept moving, playing games, calling friends, stuff like that.

Update

Nashawn is healthy now; his bone marrow transplant was a success. He wants to go to college and participate in all the things he missed out on during his many years of cancer treatment.

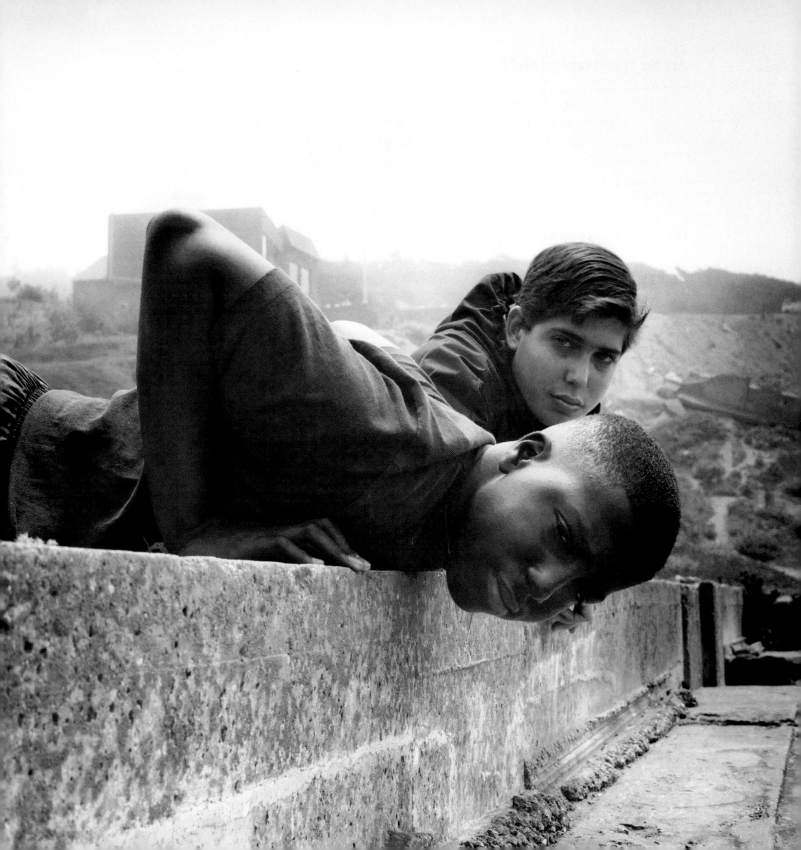

Jimmy and Antione

15 and 14 years old
Acute lymphoblastic leukemia

Antione and Jimmy attend the same teenage cancer support group in San Francisco. When I first meet them in November 1991, Antione has been getting chemotherapy treatment for a year, and Jimmy has been taking chemotherapy since his diagnosis in December 1989.

Although Antione and Jimmy come from very different cultural and economic backgrounds, they share a mutual understanding of the same disease. They both agree that they probably would never have met if they did not have cancer. However, they rarely talk about cancer and the daily trials of their treatments. Instead, they spend their time together sharing similar interests, such as sports, school, and girls.

Antione lives near San Francisco with his mother, Bettie, and his younger brother, Jermaine. Antione is in the ninth grade at a public school. Jimmy lives near the San Francisco Bay with his mother, Donna, his father, Jim, and his younger brother, Michael. He is in the tenth grade at a private school.

Jimmy and Antione are both extremely close to their families, and they tell me they have become even closer since they were diagnosed with leukemia. Antione and Jimmy both remember when they were initially very sick because of the cancer and the subsequent treatments. They are learning how to work around their treatment schedules in order to live their lives and do what they want to do, regardless of cancer.

About a month after we first met, we sit down for an interview in a local diner, comfortable talking with one another and sharing our experiences of living with cancer. In between eating, and laughter, Jimmy and Antione tell me how they are doing.

Antione (left) and
Jimmy at the beach.

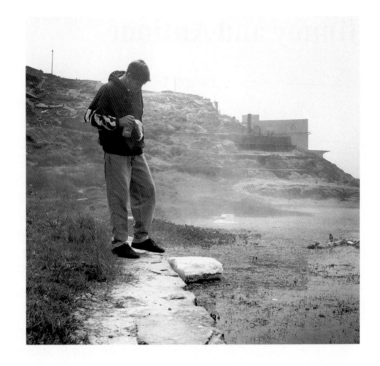

November 1991

How did you first meet, and what has it been like having cancer?

Jimmy: Antione and I go to a group for teenagers with cancer. That's where we met each other. The group meets every other week and we do all kinds of things together. We went to a '49ers' practice, we saw a Warriors' game, we went to the amusement park, Great America, we have barbecues. It's fun. We don't really talk about being sick when we're together, we just do fun things.

I guess leukemia messes up my life, but I try to adjust, to work it in. In the very beginning, it stopped my life. I went into the hospital. No school, nothing, just medicine and stuff. Then I started getting tutored and catching up with my schoolwork. I didn't have to miss a grade. My teachers were pretty helpful; they came to the hospital to help me.

Antione: I'm not going to play basketball this year. If I was able to play, I think I'd be too tired. We had tryouts, and for, like, ten minutes I was

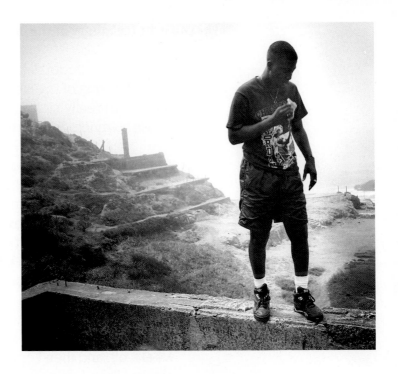

running up and down the court. I was so tired and breathing so hard that I had to lay down. I just couldn't catch my breath. I don't want to play on the team and then have something happen to me. I don't want to be a weak man on the court.

Jimmy: Before I knew I was sick, I was playing basketball and I was really tired. I was on two teams at the same time, and I told the coach I had to quit one of them. He was yelling at me for not hustling as much as I should have. I don't play anymore, but the doctors tell me I can do whatever I can handle. If my blood counts are low, like under 500, then I can't do nothing. But if my blood counts go higher and I'm feeling good, then I can do what I want.

Antione: When I have a low blood count I can't even go to the movies. I can't go out. Nothing. The doctor takes my counts about every week. Five hundred is right on the line, and I can't do anything until they come up. Sometimes that takes a week. The doctors have a schedule, and they tell me when they think my blood counts are going to go down.

67

Do you ever feel angry at the doctors because you're sick?

Jimmy: No. I understand. My doctor is always trying his hardest not to get in the way of my life. I try not to stop myself from doing anything unless I'm really sick. I try to go to school as much as possible because I miss so much. But if I'm really not feeling good, I don't go.

Antione: Sometimes I just be really tired. This morning I didn't want to get up. I just laid in the bed and laid in the bed and laid in the bed. My mom said, "Is this a sign you're not going to school today?" I went, but it was only so I didn't have to write a report for gym. My gym teacher makes us write a report about a sports player every day you are out of class. It's so stupid, she knows I'm sick. Some days I don't want to go but I know I have to because of her.

Jimmy: I have a pretty tough maintenance schedule. I'm on a two-month cycle, so I get Cytoxan in the beginning of the month, then I get two weeks off, and then I come in for vincristine every week for, like, three weeks. Then I come in for methotrexate, then I have a two-week break, then I get adriamycin and Ara-C, then a break and Cytoxan again. Some of the drugs make me sick, some don't. I think Ara-C is the worst. It's a shot that makes me really nauseous. I get my medicine after school. Sometimes I miss school the next day.

Some of my close friends know I'm sick, but not everybody. You can't really tell from looking at me. I don't really talk about it too much with them. I'll say I can't do something because I've got to go to chemotherapy. And they say alright. One of my friends jokes about it. I'll say I can't come to school for a week because my counts are low, and he'll say, "Oh yeah, my counts are down too!" I never talk seriously about it. I don't want to think about it. I've got to go into the hospital this weekend for Cytoxan. I've got to go in early so I can get hydrated [fluids]. They can't give it to me if I don't have enough fluid in my body. If I drink before I go into the hospital, it makes it easier.

Antione: Man, you've got a hard maintenance! I hate drinking so much. I'm peeing all night. All night.

What would you tell other teenagers to help them get through treatments?

Antione: Don't think about it. I try not to and that helps me. If you think about it you get depressed. I used to get depressed a lot. I don't now because I'm almost done with the hard stuff. My maintenance will be real easy. I start soon.

Jimmy: That's so easy. That's it? That's all you're taking? I have to go in to the hospital all the time for my chemotherapy. I've been in the hospital, I don't know, like, over twenty times.

When you date, do you tell girls you're sick?

Jimmy: I don't really care. When I told my friend Heather, she kind of tripped out. It was a big surprise for her. She started, like, looking up all these books, wrote an eight-page report on leukemia and stuff. It didn't

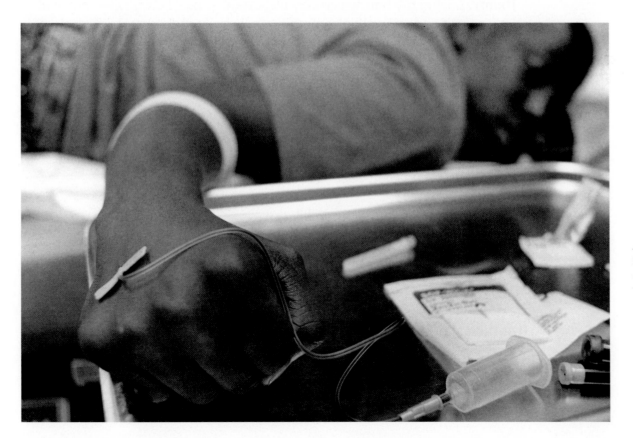

Antione
receiving
chemotherapy
through an IV.

bother me. I was a little flattered, in fact. If I have a situation where I have to bring it up, I will. But if I don't have to, I don't. Most of the time I don't really want to say it.

Antione: I've lost my hair three different times. At first I cut it off. Then I had radiation, and that took out what had grown back. Then I was bald. Then it came back real nice, but during the summer I had to go into the hospital for chemotherapy, and it fell out again. Those drugs don't let you keep your hair. It depresses me when it comes out. I'd be mad 'cause I don't like my hair to fall out. Nothing to do about it. We're not allowed to wear hats in school, but I wear mine. Sometimes people ask me, "How do you get permission to wear a hat in school?" I say, "I don't know. I guess I'm special." But I say it in a sarcastic way so nobody asks me about it. Now my hair's growing back, so it doesn't really make a difference. I don't have to wear a hat, anyway.

Jimmy: Losing my hair was really important to me. I didn't like that at all. I felt so self-conscious. It's something that really makes you different. Something physical that changes you. In the beginning, when I found out my hair was going to fall out, I was totally bummed. That was really bad. Luckily, I only lost it for two months and then I wore an Arabic bandanna.

Antione: It seems easier for me being black. When you see a white person walking down the street bald it looks kind of funny. But when you see a black person bald-headed, I don't know, it's different. A lot of black people wear their hair really low. It doesn't look so funny.

What is the worst part about being sick?

Jimmy: I don't know. I try to make it a separate part of my life. I do everything I want, and if that gets in the way sometimes, then it's alright. The Ara-C and Cytoxan aren't so great. They make me throw up.

Antione: For some reason, the medicine doesn't make me throw up. Jimmy gets sick from a lot of the stuff. When I take that antinausea stuff, zofran, I don't get sick. I feel fine. I don't know why that is, especially 'cause my dosage is so high. I usually get two asparaginase shots compared to one, which most kids get. I've had to get them in both legs. I

70

get wheezy just thinking about it. My mom gives it to me at home. Sometimes you get a knot in your leg in the muscle where you got to get the shot. That hurts. When they push the medicine in, the knot sometimes starts to grow. I'm not even going to think about it. It makes me sick.

Jimmy: After that shot of Ara-C, I can't move my leg for, like, ten minutes. It hurts so much, and it makes me nauseous. I think that's the worst part of my chemotherapy. You have to put ice on your leg first to numb where the shot is going to be.

Antione: I used to do that, and now I'm, like, scared to touch ice in the refrigerator. I'm serious. When I go get ice to put in my glass, I pick it up with a napkin. I'm telling you, I do not like ice. You know when you take an ice tray and break it to get ice? I can't even do that. My mom can tell you, I don't like ice at all. I hate ice. I'm scared of it. From the shot. Oooh . . . no ice. No ice. Oh, my God. . . .

I hate it when the doctors stink. Then I go home after my treatment and I smell just like the hospital. Man, I don't like that. Every day when I come home from the hospital I smell like some medicine. I gotta hop in the shower, then I feel better.

Jimmy: When I'm in the hospital, I just try not to do anything. I'm pretty much just there for the chemotherapy. I watch movies. I don't even get too much of my homework done. I just kind of space out.

Antione: I just play Nintendo and watch TV. I don't do anything else. At my hospital, they got Nintendo and hundreds of movies. When I was at my old hospital, the nurses always came in and talked to me. Sometimes they'd bring me back food from the cafeteria, or they'd go to McDonald's for me. One person would go out and get food for everybody.

Jimmy: I could never eat McDonald's or something when I'm in the hospital. I'd get so sick. I can't eat if I'm sick from the drugs. In the induction [the first phase of chemotherapy] I lost thirty pounds. Then I brought it back up, and I've been staying at this weight through maintenance. I get prednisone, a steroid too, for a period of a week. Prednisone has an accumulative effect. It takes a while for it to build up. But eventually it makes you hungry. I kind of get chubby cheeks from it. I heard some real horror

71

stories from people about how moody it can make you. I don't really get that moody. It's hard to tell if you're the one being moody 'cause you think you've got your reasons.

What are your relationships with your parents like?

Antione: I'd say my relationship with my mom is better now. Sometimes I take out my anger on her. Sometimes I take it out on my little brother. I just yell mostly. My little brother comes in and messes with me all the time. That's when I lose it. Like I'll be sitting there watching TV, and he'll come in singing and dancing. I'll just want to be left alone, and he'll want to mess around. Then my mom will want me to do something, and I'll really get mad 'cause I don't want to do it. Oh, man . . . they pick the wrong times to mess with me, always.

Jimmy: My mom pretty much lets me do what I want. I spend a lot more time with her now. I didn't used to talk to her much. Now we're closer. I'm pretty glad about that. My dad is very different than my mom. He wants me to follow all the things the doctors say to the dime and be very careful. I'm never supposed to drink out of anyone's soda or anything like that. I don't know. I don't think I'm angry at my parents or anything. I've just kind of accepted being sick. I don't take it out on or resent anyone.

I sometimes get mad at my little brother, but our relationship is about the same. We get along pretty well, we always did. When I'm sick he tries to do stuff for me 'cause he feels bad. He'll, like, buy me a tape or something. But that was more in the beginning. Now, when I get a game or a present, he'll try to take it out of my hands.

Antione: My brother's younger than Jimmy's. He didn't take my getting sick too well. He was only 8 when it happened. He thought I was going to die. Before, he would always say, "I wish you were dead. I wish you weren't my brother." Then, when I got sick, he'd come into the hospital crying, saying he didn't wish I was dead. It made me feel kind of good that my brother loves me. I told him it was alright, I wasn't going to die. Now he says, "You got leukemia. You gotta get a shot in your bootie." I just laugh.

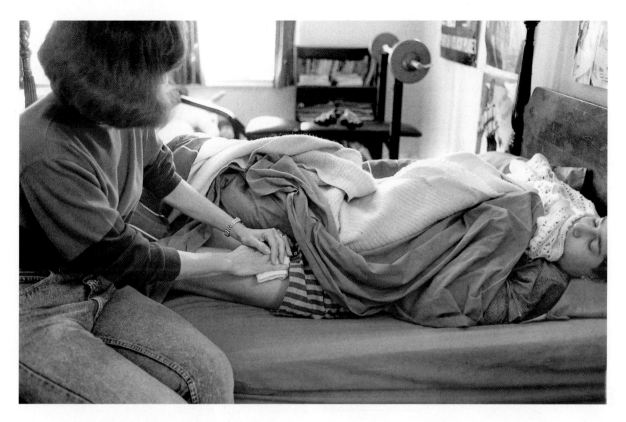

Jimmy's mom, Donna, prepares his leg for a chemotherapy shot by numbing it with ice to minimize the pain. She gives Jimmy a shot as part of his home care.

I don't know about my mom. Last time we went to the hospital my girlfriend came with us. When we dropped her off, my mom wanted to know if I really liked her. Come on! Leave me alone!

Jimmy: My mom does the exact same thing! She always tries to find out who I'm talking to on the phone and stuff. Then when we're in the car she says, "Just tell me one thing, do you like that girl?" Man! It's pretty much all about girls.

Antione: My mom says, "If you're thinking about doing anything and she's scared to go to her mom, she can come to me." I'm like, "Mom . . . ," but she's pretty open. I think that's good.

Do you ever think about the positive side of having cancer?

Jimmy: I try to, but there aren't too many advantages. I mean, occasionally I get to miss a test or something. In the beginning I got lots of cards and presents. We had, like, three or four shopping bags full of cards, but then it kind of died down. When I first came back from being sick, everyone at my school knew who I was, even all the little kids. I was like a hero. People I didn't even know were coming up to me.

Antione: That's the same with me. When I came back, everybody knew I was in the hospital. This is my first year at the new high school. I always try to make friends with everybody. I don't have no enemies. A lot of people like my girlfriend, but she's my girl.

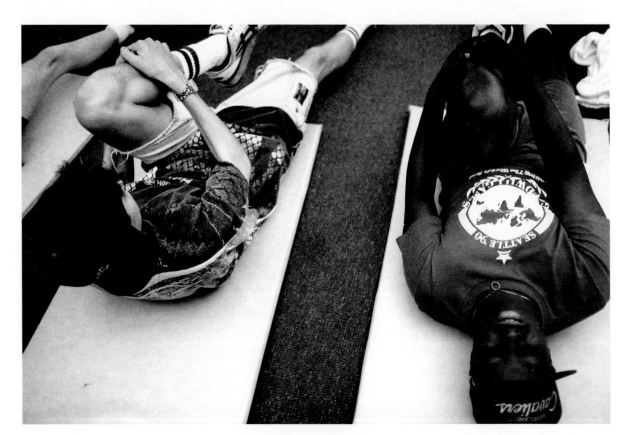

Jimmy and Antione at the gym.

Do you feel that being sick has changed your life?

Jimmy: It's hard to notice changes when you're going through them, especially when it's such a long treatment period. Sometimes I wonder what I'd be like if I never had to go through this. I think I have, pretty much, a normal teenage life. I don't feel that I've missed too much. I really try to keep my life up, stay active. It's important to me.

Right now I'm involved in crew. I'm also directing a program at my school where we work with the Ronald McDonald House. We do stuff on the holidays, decorate, bring food, make entertainment. And I'm doing something at school with a senior guy called "School after School." That's where we get student teachers to teach accelerated public school elementary kids. If I hadn't gotten sick, I wouldn't have gotten into all these nonsport things. I like what I do now, it's changed me a lot actually. I'd rather never have gotten sick, but I think I'm a better person. I can see the advantages of the person I've become as a result of all this.

Antione: I wouldn't be sitting here if I never got sick. I would never have met Jimmy or a lot of new people I've met. I just hate to go to the doctor's. I missed out on a lot of things, but I hope I can make up what I missed out on. I say that if I can make the basketball team with leukemia on heavy doses of medicine then I can do just about anything. I feel like I've accomplished a lot.

October 1991

I had talked on the phone with Antione's mother, Bettie, several times before we finally meet. She is open and friendly as we sit down in her living room to talk about her experiences as a mother whose son is in the midst of cancer treatments. Antione also joins in the conversation.

Antione
Bettie, Antione's mother

How has the cancer affected your lives?

Bettie: Antione doesn't say it anymore, but he used to tell me he wanted to hit something. He wanted to hit the wall, punch anything. He was very angry about his diagnosis. His main question was, "Am I going to live?" At the time, the doctors couldn't give him any guarantees.

They began chemotherapy treatments, and Antione went into remission right away. He was especially angry with me, but with everyone else he was fine. It was like the major attack on Mom. I know I'm always badgering him: "How do you feel? Can't you tell me what's going on? Have you taken your medicine?" But I look at him now, and I really see growth since this all began a year ago.

Antione: I've been getting treatments now for almost a year. I was diagnosed November 10th of 1990. When they first put me on chemotherapy they didn't know I would have to have such heavy doses. I get three times the normal amount because I have a chromosome deficiency. Not many kids have this.

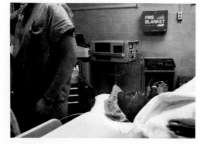

Antione is in the operating room, waiting to have his Port-a-Cath removed.

Bettie: Before he got sick he was really run down. I'd come in from work on the weekend and he'd be stretched out, lifeless. I didn't know what the problem was. He didn't want to do his chores. It was a few weeks before I really noticed that Antione didn't look right. I thought, "It's the flu. I can deal with it. I'm not paranoid." Then, out of the blue, he came home with this fever, 104.5 degrees. I took him to the doctor and they told us it was just the flu. Take Tylenol, they said. Two days later the fever was back. They put him on antibiotics. A few weeks later he complained about stomach pains, bad diarrhea. He just felt terrible. In retrospect, I encourage parents to take more caution. Don't assume a cold is a cold. Don't ignore things. You really need to be aware.

Antione was a major basketball player for his school. One night he had a basketball game, and he could barely make it through. He would run down the court and just wait for the ball to come to him. As soon as the game was over he said he was hungry and he wanted to go home. As a mother, there is a part of you that says, "Fine, we'll deal with this at home if you want to." But the other part of me said, "No, I'm winning this fight, we're going to the doctor." That night we waited in the emergency room for a couple of hours, and I told the doctor to run every test possible. The nurse came in and told me they wanted to keep him to run more tests. I didn't ever think they would say it was leukemia.

When I came back the next day they told me they were transferring him to another hospital because they were full. They told me the ambulance was on the way. I wanted to stay calm, but I was thinking, "Ambulance? Specialist?" I will never forget when Antione said to me, "Mom, I know they don't know what's wrong with me, but I hope I don't have some stupid disease." I said, "Antione, you have the flu. It's no big deal. They'll keep you. They'll give you some medicine. You'll be back at home in no time doing the same stuff."

After we found out he had cancer, we met a lot of people real fast. A lot of doctors. After a couple of weeks we got used to it. I don't think I'd met anyone at that hospital who was not loving and caring and concerned and trying to do their very best. They wanted us to know everything that was going on with him. That has made it easier for us. At first, Antione spent thirteen days in the hospital. He went through surgery to have his Port-a-Cath put in. They did a bone marrow test and told me that if he hadn't come in he'd only have lived about three more months.

I've learned a lot about this child. You spend a lot of time with a person, you get close, you fight a lot, and you learn a lot. Antione was pretty quiet through all of it, especially when the doctors were telling us what was going on. He lay there, he didn't scream out or anything. He had some tears. And I just sort of sat there and listened to what they told us we'd have to do and started to make decisions.

I'm not a crybaby. I'm not the type to fall apart at the seams. After spending time at the hospital the nurses were saying, "You are the calmest mom. Are you sure you want to watch what's happening?" I saw everything with the exception of the Port-a-Cath operation. There was nothing they did that I didn't want to see.

One day the psychologist and I were talking, and I thought, "I'm not crying. Am I *supposed* to cry? How am I *supposed* to feel?" You really don't know how you're supposed to react. You know there is not a whole lot you can do, but you should try to stay in control of what you can.

How did you feel when they first told you that you had leukemia?

Antione: I didn't know what it was, but I thought I was going to die, and I didn't even really begin my life yet. I knew there wasn't too much I could do, so I decided I would just do my best. I thought maybe God wanted me to look at my life as it is and appreciate what I have. I was angry, though. I didn't show it when the doctors were there, just to my mom. I cried a little bit. Before the Port-a-Cath operation, I'd never been in surgery before. I wasn't too scared. The doctors said I took the news better than a lot of other kids. I take the pain better, too. I have a high tolerance for it.

Bettie: Antione doesn't miss much school. The doctors are amazed he gets there as much as he does because he's getting a triple dose of chemotherapy. I'm really proud of him for pushing, but I tell him not to go too far. He's still playing basketball, even with his prednisone cheeks.

We recently had to transfer back to our original hospital. It was a big deal for Antione, and it's very different. We went into a room, and the doctor laid Antione on a bare table. No sheet. He had the chemo drugs in his hands, and he opened the miniblinds above. Those blinds gather a lot of dust, but the doctor just wiped off his Port and gave him his chemo. I was sitting there with my mouth open. It's not like I could complain about it. I had no choice. I either had to come back to the hospital or get a new insurance carrier. That wasn't an option.

This is how it is. I believe you have to adjust to certain things that happen in your life. You've got to get around them. They still give chemo the same way, they're just totally different in their approach. It's almost like the difference between the Hilton and a Motel 6.

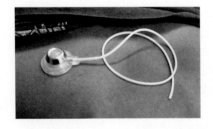

A Port-a-Cath before it is inserted into the upper chest.

Antione: I just go day by day. It's hard to go to school sometimes. I get tired, especially with the heavy doses of chemo I'm getting. Pretty soon I'll be going on a maintenance schedule, so I'll be going to school more often and to the hospi ʰl less. I try not to think too much about it. I go to the doctor's, I go to s   I do what I have to do to keep up with everything.

I had a tutor for a while. I also had to go to summer school. It really doesn't matter to me if the kids at school know I'm sick. Now that I'm in a big new high school, not many people know. Last year, at my old school, everybody knew. What can I do? They can't catch it; they just think I don't come to school as much as I should.

Bettie: I think this disease is devastating to brothers and sisters. His brother, Jermaine, is better now, but he went through a lot emotionally. He wanted to die. He wanted to take chemo. He came with us once to the hospital, and Antione got sick from the drugs. Antione started to throw up, and Jermaine got very upset. I didn't see a lot of crying, mostly fighting. They're siblings, but they're angry. I have to explain a lot. Jermaine feels left out. He thinks he's not as important. He thinks I don't love him as much as Antione. Jermaine says, "Antione gets special things, he gets more clothes, he gets this, he gets that," on and on.

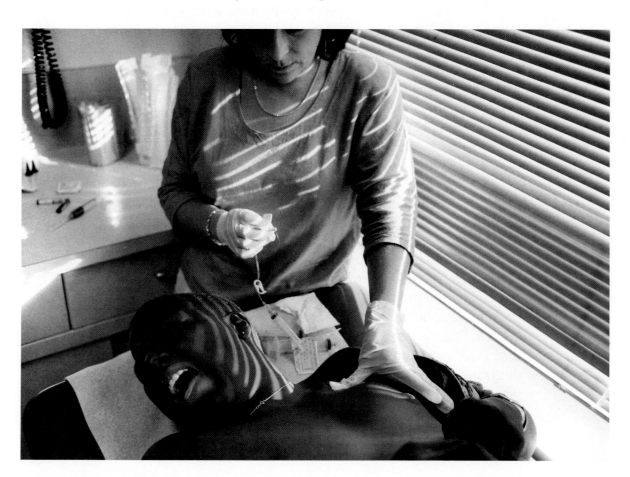

Antione gets his Port-a-Cath cleaned by a nurse, a procedure that can be painful.

I do have to do more for the one who is sick. It's not that I do it intentionally. As a single parent, I pray for the single parents who want to fall apart. I remember thinking, "He's on the couch, he's sick, he's throwing up. I put him in my room with some soda and the television, some special attention." One is screaming from one room and the other from the other room. I thought I'd go crazy.

Jermaine actually went to the hospital for a siblings day. They showed them a film, they talked, looked at pictures. Then he went to siblings camp. He loved it. I planned some nice things for Antione and I to do when Jermaine was away. We wanted to go out to dinner, to the movies. We wanted to have fun, but Antione got sick. He got a fever, neutropenia [low white blood-cell count], and had to be in the hospital for seven days. That was the end of that fun.

When I picked Jermaine up from camp he came over to the car and said, "Mom, I loved it so much I want to come back tomorrow." Antione didn't want to go at all. I think he had it in his mind that everyone was being pushed around in wheelchairs, sick, with tubes coming out of their stomachs. It's really for kids who have been sick and are getting over it, or who just love it so much they keep coming back even after their treatments are over. I picked Antione up after camp was over and he said, "Mom, I loved it so much I can't wait to come back." He had a wonderful time.

Antione: Me and Jimmy went to camp together. We didn't want to go at first. We decided to go, and it was fun. We did all kinds of things. We went hiking, had parties, played sports,archery, water-skied, met lots of people. We weren't supposed to think about being sick. We just had fun.

Life is kind of hard now. I lost my hair twice, and I think I'll lose it probably one more time. It grows back fast. Once I get through this last month in the hospital and go on maintenance, I think life will be much easier. Sometimes I can't do things I really want to do. I can't play basketball because I don't have the energy, and I've missed out on a lot of stuff like time with my friends, and parties. The doctors try to work my chemo around stuff I want to do. They didn't want me sad all the time. Through the hospital I heard about Make-a-Wish. Me, my mother, my brother, and my best friend are going to Hawaii for Christmas for a week. Everything is included—the plane, food, hotel. I need it.

Hanging out with my friends helps me a lot, especially the ones who have cancer or have had it. The support group helps, too. We tell how we feel, and we do all kinds of things together like eat, go to movies, go skiing. We don't focus on being sick, but we do talk about it. We take a few minutes out of the group to tell what's going on. It makes it much easier to have somebody to relate to. At first I didn't have nobody to relate to. But now I have a lot of friends who I can talk to, a lot of people I probably wouldn't have met if I wasn't sick.

Bettie: Antione is on steroids, but he's begun tapering down. He was taking eighteen milligrams, but he'll be down to eight. The first time he took steroids he gained over twenty pounds. This time, and the last, he was very careful about what he ate. Mind over matter. He knew he had no control over the hunger that goes along with the steroids. Everything reminded him of food. I think as you get more and more into the disease you learn about what you have control over, and you work on it.

Also, Antione had an allergic reaction to the asparaginase shot. His body reacted like a diabetic's, and he had to have insulin for a month and a half. We came home not only with syringes for Ara-C but a schedule for insulin and all sorts of instructions. Antione had to carry a little blood monitor around with him and give himself shots every day.

In the beginning Antione was very, very sick. We were kind of afraid to talk about it. Now during the course of a few weeks, he'll feel nauseous and want to throw up. For me, that was so difficult, watching a person throw up so much that the lining of the stomach is coming out. He threw up until there was nothing more. It took some time for me to adjust to that, and it seems he's adjusted to it, too. Maybe Antione's building up a tolerance. Some drugs he's taking now would have made him feel deathly ill a few months ago.

Antione: In the beginning I really felt like my whole life had changed. At first I wondered what I ever did to get sick. Why me? I was really angry. My mom said it's something I have to live with. My uncle said that by getting it, it would make me a better man in life. That's how I try to look at it. I try not to look at it like the world owes me something because I have it. It's really nobody's fault. I've been thinking that someday, when it's all over, I'd like to take time out of my life to help other kids.

January 1992

Donna and I had talked on the phone several times before we first meet at the hospital where Jimmy is getting his Cytoxan, a chemotherapy drug that requires a hospital stay. We visit downstairs in the cafeteria while Jimmy rests in his hospital room. Most of the time when Jimmy is in the hospital, Donna stays with him, sleeping on a chair in his room.

Donna, Jimmy's mother

In the beginning, Jimmy was so sick for so long. In retrospect, we know it was the chemotherapy. It was just particularly hard on him. At the time, it was more of a mystery to us. He missed most of the last half of his eighth-grade year and was either at home or in the hospital. It was really a tough time for us. We really had to learn what leukemia was. Leukemia to us was cancer, and something you die from. We didn't know that the recovery rate was so high. It takes a while to understand all that.

I think back on what we've all gone through these last few years of Jimmy's treatments for leukemia, and I'm so relieved that I was in the position to have time off to be with him. My husband and I work together in a family-owned business, so I started working half-time when he got sick. I think it would be so much harder on Jimmy if I couldn't be with him. At least now, he knows that I'm always there. His dad and brother are there for him too, but he knows he never has to do any of this on his own, even though, obviously, he is the one getting treatment.

Jimmy's treatment plan is so aggressive. If I can help make his life easier so he doesn't have to miss out on much, he can put more into his life right now. I will drive him to school and pick him up. I'll drive him to the clinic or to sports practice and make sure he has a ride home. I do those things so Jimmy doesn't have to worry about them.

What we're going through right now bears no resemblance to the early stages of leukemia treatment two years ago. Jimmy really is so much more stable now. There is a certain rhythm to his treatments now, and we know what to expect, what it's going to be like. He's been fortunate enough to have his blood counts rebound every time, so we've been able to stay on schedule. Jimmy hasn't missed any of his chemotherapy. It's actually pretty easy now. His entire treatment plan is for

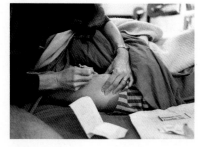

Jimmy's mother gives him a chemotherapy shot at home.

three years, two months. He had a month of induction, a month of consolidation, then he has eighteen two-month cycles that make up his maintenance period.

Induction is supposed to be the most intensive part of the treatment. That's when they took Jimmy's blood counts down to nothing. When he was first diagnosed, he went right into the hospital and stayed there through the entire induction phase. He had very heavy doses of chemotherapy, which were meant to wipe out every living cell, good and bad, in his body. They really wiped him out. Jimmy was very susceptible to infection, and he had lots of blood transfusions.

Consolidation occurs during the second month. It's supposed to be slightly easier. A lot of that phase can be passed in the outpatient clinic. Maintenance is the next three years and should be when your life returns somewhat to normal. Jimmy got very sick during his induction and could not handle his drugs at all. He had severe headaches that lasted weeks. He had to get MRIs and other tests, too. He was vomiting and nauseous. Some of the drugs were given through the outpatient clinic. We'd go in and he'd have to lie down on the floor because there was no other place for him, and he could barely make it to get up and get the treatments.

A couple of times Jimmy had to go back in the hospital, once because he became dehydrated and once because of an infection. He continued to be so sick, and nobody could understand it. His stomach lining was totally torn apart. We tried all kinds of things to make him feel better. Throughout all of this, they never stopped the chemotherapy. They wouldn't delay it. Jimmy went from 130 to 111 pounds, which is most of his body fat. In the hospital, they put in a temporary tube to feed him.

My husband took it really hard. I was more geared toward helping Jimmy get through it. Later, we traded off emotions. Nothing can compare to the possible loss of your child. Nothing can knock you off the structure you thought you had in your life. We don't feel that way anymore, luckily. Jimmy was diagnosed high-risk leukemia because of his age and symptoms. He just passed the two-year mark since diagnosis, so that puts him back with everybody else with leukemia. He's not high-risk anymore. We've been seeing Jimmy's body respond well to the drugs now. He's bounced back. He's gone from 111 to 152 pounds now. He's also grown and gotten stronger and is doing everything he wants. It's so much easier than it was. Jimmy has been hitting certain benchmarks, like the two-year mark, and moving right along. Now, for us, understanding the disease as we do, we can proceed with our lives.

When we first learned about the leukemia we did just about everything. This hospital is pretty good about providing information. We met with all of his doctors and had about a two-hour session on leukemia, on Jimmy's diagnosis, and what was going to happen to him on the chemotherapy. We taped the entire meeting. The hospital also has two oncology nurses on staff, and we had a meeting with them, too. We talked about what was going on in childhood cancer, dealing with everything from nutrition to side effects to administering drugs. We also talked to another parent whose son had been diagnosed two years before Jimmy. They were really terrific about meeting with us, discussing their experiences and what we could expect.

My husband, Jim, also spent a lot of time at the hospital, in the library. They have a system where you can make very specific inquiries and call up to get information about what's going on in terms of research. You can also get copies of articles. We just tried to fill in the missing pieces with all of that. Sometimes the articles would be misleading and sometimes correct. A lot of the library research was out of date, so we had to make sure we didn't go back too far, or it could be scary. But I've found that the things that are most descriptive are scary. We just tried to stay on top of it.

At this point, I'm interested in long-term effects and in studies that discuss shortening maintenance periods. Unfortunately, that's not going to happen in Jimmy's time. When Jimmy was first diagnosed, we were given a choice of maintenance programs. He could have been treated on the New York plan, which is what he is on, which has a very tough maintenance program. He has a three-day period where he gets Ara-C, a drug that is very hard on him. I actually give him the shot at home, every twelve hours for three days. It makes him very sick. He also gets intravenous methotrexate, which is a four-hour infusion, every two months. He gets about three or four other drugs, either orally or he'll come in to the hospital for them. It's a very aggressive program.

The German program, which appeared to be an alternative at that point, was probably more aggressive up front. You have something called a reconsolidation, where you go back in after two months and they hit you hard again after the consolidation phase. After that, the three-year

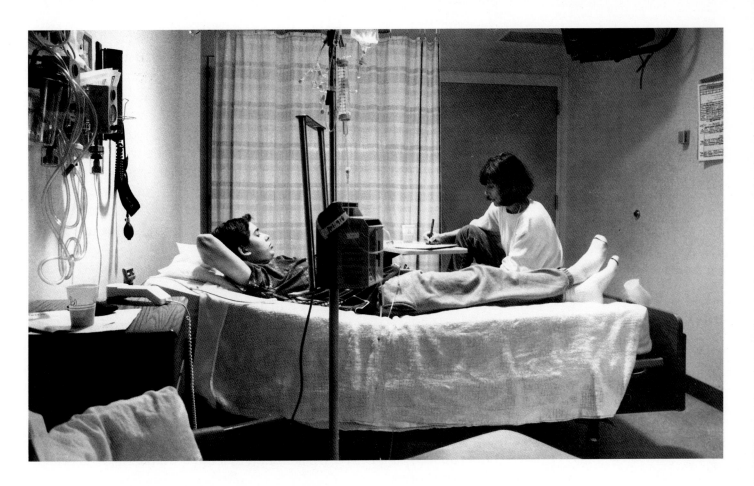

maintenance period is relatively easy. You go in the clinic infrequently, and none of the drugs are too strong.

    As intelligent or as naive as you might be, you really have to sort through a tremendous amount of information very, very quickly. The parent isn't capable of fully understanding most decisions that are being made. You want to understand the treatment plan, but at the same time, you're going through the anguish of possibly losing your child, who is very sick and can't hold his head up by himself. He can't move. He can't get out of a horizontal position. You combine all these things, the risk, the pain, and the responsibility of making sure your child is getting the best care and the right treatment.

    We're very lucky to have wonderful doctors here, and to be so close and so confident in this institution. The hospital itself could improve

Jimmy and his mother review schoolwork while he undergoes chemotherapy in the hospital.

85

its patient care—I've been involved in that lately—but the medical care is tremendous. A few parents and I have been involved in improving the environment for the patients. We wanted to divide the rooms so teenagers wouldn't be sleeping with infants. We're trying to make the admitting process flow more smoothly. We would always have to wait for hours, even though we come in every month. And the rooms would never be ready when we would finally reach the floor. The nurses wouldn't be assigned a room, so we'd have to wait longer. The whole process could take three to twelve hours just to get Jimmy hooked up and hydrated, and he hadn't even started his chemotherapy yet. These are the things we're working on, and the hospital has been responsive to us. Things are changing for the better.

Everyone talks about learning the tricks of the experienced hospital patient, such as getting the urinal so you can start collecting the urine. Getting to know someone so they can tuck you away where you are more comfortable. But you know, when you're at your worst, in the early stages, you don't know stuff like that. You don't know anything.

I can look back now and wonder why I even cared about all those little things. They are not important in the big picture. The fact is that Jimmy is getting better. He's got good medical care. I can put the little things in perspective, but nevertheless, when you're in it on a daily basis, when you come back repeatedly and the same things are happening, it becomes unacceptable. We are shocked that the administration is listening to our concerns.

Our oncology nurse is incredible. She's dedicated and gives us most of our information. A lot of the assistance and the training has come from her. She's the one who taught me how to give Jimmy the Ara-C shots, sitting with me as I practiced giving a shot to an orange. She made sure the angle was right and that I was giving the proper amount of pressure. I really appreciate all that.

I call the Ara-C Jimmy's worst drug. Most parents are trained to give the shots themselves, at home. It doesn't go into the vein, it goes into the muscle at an angle, and it's very painful. At least it's one that's easy to do, and you can't screw up. I cleanse the area and put ice on it for ten minutes and then give Jimmy the shot. It bothered me a lot at first, especially because he would get so sick after the shot. I felt like I was the one making my kid sick, even though I know I'm helping to make him better. I also didn't feel so confident that I was doing it correctly because I know

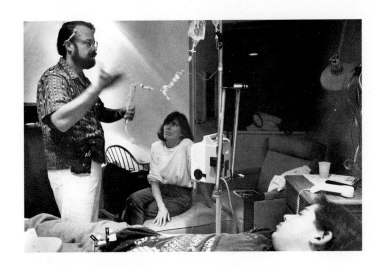

Jimmy and his mother watch the nurse set up the chemotherapy IV.

that the speed that I push the needle can cause more pain or less pain. It just was a matter of getting it down. Right now I feel like I'm giving the shot as best as I can. I hold the ice on his leg for ten minutes, really hard. I push slowly. I try to have him watching TV or something that distracts him.

Throughout Jimmy's illness it has been helpful to talk to other parents, especially early on. It was really good to get an idea of how other people handled things. You can get a lot of medical input even through other parents. They can tell you what they've tried for side effects, what medication they've used, what kinds of foods have helped, etc. That's all been helpful. I do go to a cancer support group at least once a month. There are some other parents there who have teenagers who are sick, so the support relating to teen issues is there. The group helps me to remember that other people have dealt with Ara-C shots or similar things. Within the group there are a lot of answers, a lot of help available.

Cancer is hard on families. Jim and I have been lucky in the sense that this happened at a stage in our lives when we didn't have other extreme demands. We've had the flexibility in our home life not to be stretched to the absolute limit. Regardless, it's hard. There is just no getting around that. Having friends who can help is really important. We had so many people step forward unexpectedly.

In the beginning, Jimmy had to have massive blood transfusions. Thirty or forty, I don't even know. We wanted it all to be from donors we knew. All the donors had to be free from a certain kind of infection and antibody, then they had to be matched to Jimmy's blood type. We had a group of friends who got seventy or eighty people we knew to come to the hospital to be tested, and of those, thirty could be donors. They all gave blood at least once. It was a tremendous relief to us knowing whose blood Jimmy was going to use. Hepatitis can be a risk. Jimmy was so weak we just wanted to know where the blood was coming from.

Other things from friends helped: delivering food, bringing over dinner, being there. My folks live here in California, and that helped. When Jimmy was diagnosed, my mother stayed at home and helped out. She also relieved me when I needed to be away from the hospital. We were lucky. Other people would call later and say, "We didn't call you because we didn't know what to say." Well, there were certainly times when I didn't want to take any phone calls, but I did. It shouldn't work that way. Someone should at least be able to come up with something to say. We've had our share of instances where people have said things that were incredibly dumb. That doesn't really matter, it's just important for people to stand by you.

Although we don't always admit to it, parents really do need help. Everyone calls and asks what they can do. Usually I tell them I appreciate it, but I don't need anything. It's kind of a good idea to think of things they can do, especially if you are going through a long illness. Someone can always do an errand, pick up something to eat, return the movies to the video store. I can't say that I did that much of it, but it's a good idea. It makes them feel good, too.

My younger son, Michael, has been basically pretty attentive to Jimmy, especially earlier on, but he still maintains his sibling independence. They fight occasionally. Michael actually did really well, he didn't treat Jimmy as if he were going to die. He was OK, yet he would sit down and have serious questions about what was happening to his brother. We tried not to act terribly frightened in front of Michael, but we tried to tell him, as we did with Jimmy, the truth. We were perfectly honest with them, although we didn't show extreme emotions in front of them. Michael did overhear a conversation that his grandmother was having with a friend of hers back home. She was really letting it all out, and she was so upset. That kind of worried me. But Michael didn't really hear anything in the conversation that we hadn't told him. Jimmy could die, but treatments are such that kids usually make it.

I sort of like the way Michael has treated Jimmy. Even now, when Jimmy's home sick, he'll do little things, but not too much. He's still a little brother. They've struck a nice balance.

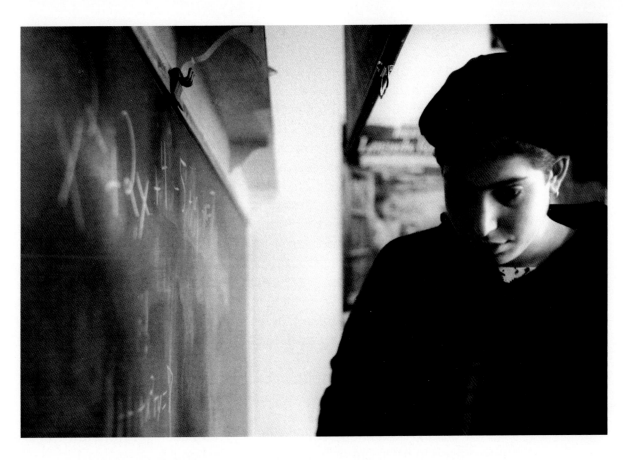

Jimmy tutors a student in math after school.

January 1992

Michael attends the same school as Jimmy, and because they are very close in age, the two brothers spend a lot of time together and know many of the same kids. Michael and I find an empty classroom one day after school and sit down to talk about his brother Jimmy. Michael is eager to talk and be involved, and I quickly learn that he is very in tune with what Jimmy's going through, as well as how others at school respond to Jimmy.

Michael, Jimmy's brother, 13 years old

Jimmy got sick right before Christmas, about two years ago. I was in seventh grade at the time. We all thought he had mono. We were hoping he didn't because we didn't want him to miss Christmas.

89

Jimmy was in the hospital, and I was sleeping in his room one night. My dad came in the room at, like, three in the morning, and I knew something was wrong. Then he told me about Jimmy. My dad told me he might lose his hair. I was upset about that. Jimmy was always a good-looking guy. I thought he might not look as good. I actually think he looks better now with his new hair.

I think my dad was very weak. He cried a lot. My mom was very strong. My parents totally reversed their roles. My dad was really in a bad mood. My mom and I tried to stay as light and as up as possible. It scared me to see my dad that first night. Once, at school, after Jimmy was diagnosed, I started crying for no reason. My mom came and picked me up. I went home and watched *Arsenio Hall.* I felt much better after that.

My dad is so defensive and serious now about leukemia. Once, I made a comment about Jimmy's cheeks. They're fatter now because of some medicine he takes. I was just joking around, but my dad got really mad at me. He takes everything that has to do with leukemia so defensively. That's not usually his way. If I comment on my brother's looks it's only to joke around.

Jimmy was really sick for three months right away. That part really got to me. I started wondering, why him? Why does this always happen to the good people and not the jerks? But I was always pretty normal about it. I didn't go to the hospital a lot. My mom and dad were always there. I used to try to cheer him up whenever I could.

I never ask Jimmy about his treatments. It really doesn't matter to me what he has or what treatments he takes or what's functioning in the blood cells. I have no idea about that. I just hope he gets better. I have realized during this time who was good to us, and what friends are good to him. Some of his friends were great to him. Some of my friends, too. They sent cards, called, made stuff. I always thought about it when someone did something nice. I could stay home by myself, but sometimes the neighbors would come over or ask me to their houses. I would do laundry or bake cookies with them. They were good to me.

Everyone always joked about my getting less attention since Jimmy got sick. Whenever a relative called they would say, "Hello, Jimmy?" and I would say, "No, it's Mike." They would just say, "Oh." I joke with my parents about favoring Jimmy, but it never hurts me. My brother has leukemia. I don't. Of course my father has to pay a little more attention to him than to me. It would be selfish of me to get upset.

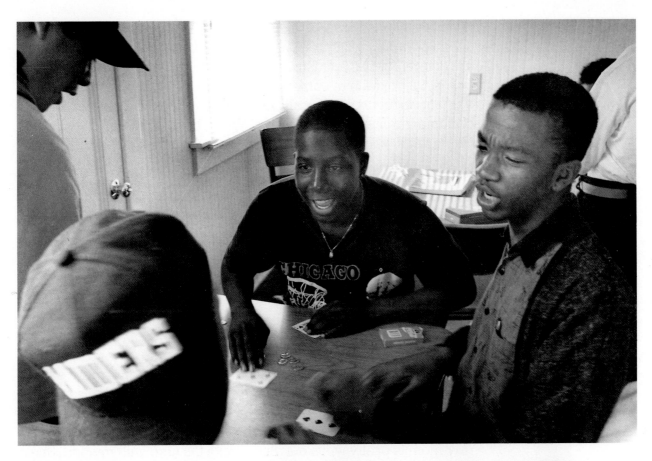

Antione jokes with his
friends while they
play cards.

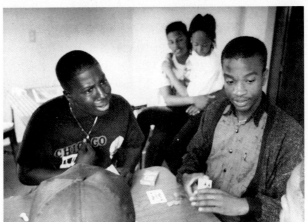

I always hang out with Jimmy when he's at home after treatments. I mean, I go on with my life, but I take care of him. When my mom and dad aren't there I get him stuff. Even if I'm outside playing basketball and he calls, I'll go get him something. We've always been close, but we never talk about things seriously. We have other things to talk about than spending our lives over leukemia. We're like a normal family, and we try to do what we normally do. Sometimes we have to check Jimmy's schedule, but we work everything around it.

I've learned a little about leukemia. It has opened my eyes to people who are suffering like this. It's made me happy to be who I am, to be healthy and stuff. I always realized it, but I don't think I should complain about my life. I always hear kids in the sixth and seventh grades complaining that their lives are so bad. I don't see why kids commit suicide and take drugs. They have healthy bodies, why waste them?

When Jimmy came back from the hospital he was really skinny, but he looks good now. I wasn't afraid of the way Jimmy looked when he came home. I really don't think he's changed at all mentally. He's still the same.

I never thought about the philosophical things about Jimmy being sick. I guess something in his body just got messed up. My dad says that he wishes it was him who got sick instead of Jimmy. I don't feel that way. I'm glad I didn't get it, but I wish he didn't either.

My mom is pretty worn out. She works full time with my dad. She works extra hours so she can take time off when my brother is sick. Then she has to come home, cook dinner, and take charge of the stuff in the house. She seems more and more worn out. I think when this leukemia thing ends she'll be able to rest. I try to help her, but I have my homework to do, and I need to practice basketball.

I think of my brother as my brother, not someone who has leukemia. I try and always be positive. I know things can go wrong, but I never think about that. I just treat him normally.

January 1992

Bettie and I have met several times since our first interview, and we are very comfortable. I have spent time with her family, going to movies, hanging out around the house, and just being with them appreciating their

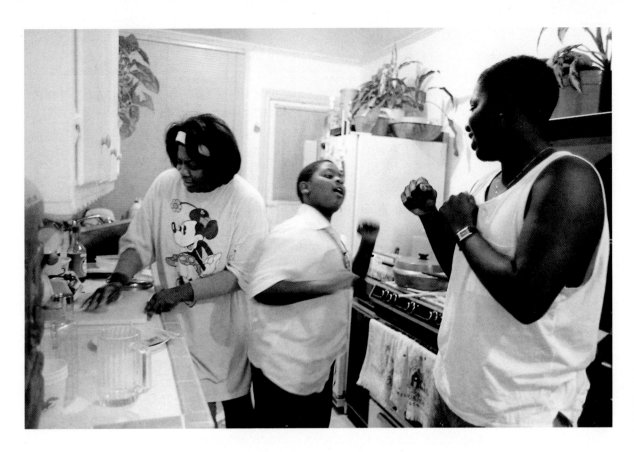

Bettie prepares dinner while Antione and his brother, Jermaine, play.

closeness and friendliness. Today, we sit down to talk about how she is doing on this journey with Antione's cancer.

Bettie, Antione's mother

At this point in time, what is your perspective on your son having cancer?

As a single mom with two kids, I have to work two jobs. I see other mothers really hurting, and they have their husbands and decent homes. I think to myself, "Maybe if they can see that I'm getting through it, and I don't even have all they do, I can help." It's great to share with the other parents who have sick children. We're all going through the same things, no matter what color you are. I also think there is a reason my child has cancer. Maybe he will make a difference.

93

I can't think of a worse thing that could have happened to us. But the best thing is that I've met so many beautiful people. There are many wonderful people outside my door that I never would have met if Antione hadn't gotten sick. I used to go to a support group, which helped. Things like a support group help make a person identify with their blessings. Everyone would love to have more. I'd love to let my kids have everything. I'd love to have someone clean my house. I'd love to have a house like Jimmy's. I'd love to change things. But you can't.

How do you think Antione is doing physically and emotionally?

Well, in the group I realized I didn't have a real sick child. Some of these children have tubes sticking into their bodies, holes in their skulls. I just have a child with a Port-a-Cath that you can't see, a bald head, and he has to go in for treatments every couple of weeks. It really made me focus.

I think it's wonderful that Antione and Jimmy are friends. They have a lot in common. It isn't all because they have the same illness. They're teenagers. They like girls. They like to do the same things, and they hang out. They both have their own set of friends, but it's funny how they both sort of linked together. They talk all the time on the phone. They went to a dance at Jimmy's school last week.

In regards to our medicine, I clearly understand that Antione is doing well. He's really fortunate that he's been in remission. As long as he stays there, with my faith—factor number one—and as long as he takes his medicine, then he should be OK.

Antione now takes medicine every day. He's taking Septra three times a week and prednisone five days each month. And he has chemo once a month and a spinal tap every three months. Things are a little more laid back now. In the beginning, I kept journals on what drugs he was taking, how he reacted. I was completely caught up. Now, I'm relaxing, and I think he is too. I'm appreciating it. It's not so traumatic. My main concern is trying to get Antione to take his medicines on time. He's been pretty good about it lately, cooperating more and remembering. It's a nuisance for him. He can always find something else to do. He's dating and he always has plans.

Do you give special attention to Jermaine now?

Yes, because I can never return the year that I snatched away from him when Antione was diagnosed. I didn't mean to ignore my child, but you have to pay attention to the one who needs you. I know Jermaine suffered a lot. He was lonely a lot. They are both latchkey kids. They have to come and go into the apartment without me being here.

Until last month, when we were going into the hospital for treatment three or four times per week, we wouldn't get home until six or seven at night. Jermaine would have been here alone for three or four hours. I began to overcompensate with food. I knew I couldn't be around for Jermaine, so I had every little treat I could possibly have for him at home. Come five o'clock, when I still wasn't home, he'd just eat it all. Now, when he's unhappy, he eats.

Jermaine's behavior has been poor. I would get calls from the school and have to go in. I got so tired of explaining to everyone the reason he was acting badly was because he was upset about his brother. Antione, though, was a complete jerk to him. He was awful. He was very demanding and angry. He was lashing out at us, because we're closest to him. He'd be fine in front of the doctor, but when he left the room, I'd be the one to get his anger.

What changes have you seen in Antione?

I'm not sure if this would have happened so soon, but I feel we've got a good relationship. I think it's because I'm such a young mom, I can be a friend, too. We've gotten to a point where I can look at him and say, "You can understand this." He's really matured a lot, and I appreciate it. This disease has forced him into that. Sometimes Antione seems so grown-up. He has to be responsible for a lot of things other children don't have to be. It's easier for us now that we're on maintenance. He can make plans, do things. I remember him sitting in the other room in the beginning, crying, saying, "Mommy, I hate this so much. I hate this so much. I can't go on. I can't do anything."

Antione, and Jimmy too, were both high-risk leukemia. They had chemo all the time. In the beginning Antione was so sick. He's really

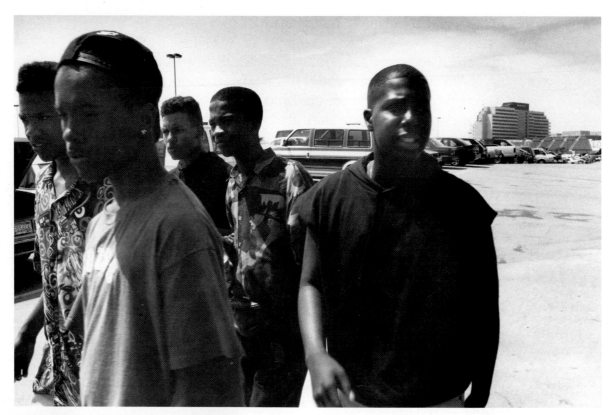

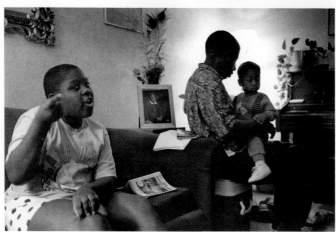

Antione (right) and his
friends on their way to
an amusement park
(top). Jermaine, 9 (left),
Antione, and his nephew
Christopher, 2.

responded to the drugs much better than anyone thought he would, especially because he gets such a high dosage because of his chromosome deficiency. One day it just seemed that his body started tolerating the drugs. He was less and less sick, more tolerant of what he had to take.

I tell Antione that I know he's having a hard time, but that he has to get beyond that. He has to recognize that the drugs make him moody and feel lousy, but at the same time he has to have respect for me and his brother. That's very important to us. We still knock heads sometimes, but I really trust Antione.

Times are hard, especially for black children. Antione sees everything that goes on in our backyard and in our front yard. We make sure we let each other know where the other is. He's very mature in that respect. I make an effort to go with him and his brother to all the movies that come out regarding drugs, gang wars, stuff like that. We go, then we talk about it. I don't want my children to go in that direction. It's scary. I really don't know what's going to happen. I just want him to be a decent man.

Do you think that having an illness has shown Antione anything positive?

I think he's more focused and confident. Realizing that he could be dead from this illness has changed his values. It's not that he didn't have them before, but this has calmed him. Before, Antione was a wild teenager.

I believe we've always been appreciative of what we've had, but just focusing on what's important to us is the major thing. Sometimes though, I get so stressed that I just run around yelling. So we decided, the three of us, no yelling, no screaming, just respect each other more. We've had a lot of pain. It's been really scary. This illness has made me really focus on my children and how important they are to me.

I think that if anyone were to say anything about Antione, they would say, ''He was really cooperative, a really good patient. He wanted whatever would cure him.'' It took Antione about seven weeks after diagnosis to focus on what they were giving him. He didn't want to know at first. He wanted me to do everything. He rebelled. Who wants to be sick at 16 years old? Now, he's very active with his sickness.

June 1992

Antione and Kisha are as close as brother and sister. They have spent all their lives together and now live in the same apartment building. They watch TV late at night, they share some of the same friends, they celebrate their birthdays together, they argue—they are family. When Antione was diagnosed, it greatly affected Kisha. She couldn't imagine the possibility of a life without her cousin Tony.

When I meet with Kisha she is packing her suitcase to leave for a special summer program for gifted students at a college in California. She is excited about her summer plans and what the future holds. Yet at the same time she is very concerned about her cousin Tony.

Kisha, Antione's cousin, 16 years old

Because Tony has leukemia, sometimes I feel bad when I get mad at him. At the same time, I want to treat him like a normal person. He was diagnosed November 10, 1990, and I still, on June 21, 1992, don't exactly know how to treat him.

We never talk about him being sick. I would always go to the hospital and stay with him. Sometimes I would spend the night. I really wanted to ask him how it felt to get that blood transfusion. He was just lying there with someone else's blood going through him. As soon as we might have talked, something else always came up.

I couldn't cry in front of him in the beginning. I wanted to so bad, especially when we were in the hospital. I could feel the tears way down in my stomach, and there was nothing I could do. I wanted to burst open and scream, ''Why? Why?''

The day we found out Tony had leukemia, I had just come home from high school. When I got home, my mother told me to sit down, she had something to tell me. She was crying. I didn't cry right away. For some reason, I felt like I didn't know enough about leukemia to burst out in tears. I ran to my encyclopedia and started reading about it. It said there were two kinds: acute and chronic. It said most younger kids acquire acute leukemia, which moves through the body quickly but is really curable. After that I told my mom what I had read, but she said that they still didn't know a lot about his condition, and maybe he could die. I was really sad. I couldn't even hold myself together.

Sometimes Tony makes me so mad I just want to strangle him, but then again, he is my cousin. I think a lot about him not getting through it. Nobody told me that his cells have been acting up recently, I had to overhear it from my mother. I couldn't imagine a life without him around. Sometimes he'll come up here and sleep on the couch, or we'll talk on the phone to friends.

At school everybody just thought, "Oh, my God, he's going to die." And then I started thinking, "This person that I've always been with isn't going to see me have kids, graduate high school, nothing." I was really going crazy. I guess now I've just learned to live with it. I know he can relapse. All this stuff runs through my mind. I don't tell people that this really, really bothers me.

I've learned that life is nothing to take for granted. One day you could be out playing basketball, and the next day you find out you may not live. I realize that there is a lot I don't know but want to know. From all this, I've learned that I want to be a cancer surgeon. It was a revelation to me. I want to teach other people about the disease. I want to share what I know. I don't even know if Tony knows what I want to do.

Tony always moves away from the subject of being sick. For me, personally, if I had leukemia, I'd be going through every library, every city looking for information. I know for a fact that I know more about his disease than he does. And that's fine because he deals better not knowing. He just listens to what the doctors tell him and that's it. He has not fallen into a deep sorrow. He has tried to keep up his normal life, and I give him a lot for that.

I definitely want to talk to him someday about how he feels. I don't want to ruin things by saying, "Hey, Tony, how do you feel about that leukemia you got?" There never seems to be a right time. If he ever dies (what a word!) I would like to have talked to him about all this. I don't want any regrets. I want to know how he felt about what he's been going through. I remember having this pathetic optimism about him. I didn't even know what was in store.

Once, I sat up there with him when he had to have a spinal tap. I watched the needle go into his spine. I thought I was going to pass out. I think I would just fall apart if that were me. Especially because he's got to take chemo for so long. I would just tell the doctors to take me and kill me right away. This is just me. Tony will go and take it all like a champ. I don't understand how.

Tony has good friends. I don't even think they trip about him being sick. It doesn't get in the way, and it's easy to forget about it now. He looks normal. Before, his face was puffy, his stomach was big. He didn't look good, especially when his hair was falling out. He looked weird. All of my friends just thought he had a bad haircut when they met him. He should feel special because he had the bald look when everybody else had the fade, and now the bald look is back in. He brought back the style.

May 1992

Antione and I talk together on a long holiday weekend. He is alone in the house, on restriction for receiving bad grades. He misses his friends and his girlfriend. He is one year and nine months into his chemotherapy and has just been told by the doctor that bad cells have been found in his spinal fluid. He doesn't seem worried. He just wants to go to his best friend, Henry's, house for a barbecue the next day.

Antione

I'm not getting along with my mom lately. We've been fighting because I'm not doing so good in school. She put me on punishment for a month. A teacher called and told her I didn't do my assignment. I didn't know I was supposed to do it. Then Monday, the doctor called and said she found some bad cells in my spinal fluid. We had to go to the hospital the next day, and that's the day the teacher called.

Now I can't go to work, I can't watch TV, I can't use the phone, I can't go outside. Can't listen to the radio either. All I can do is my home-work. My grades have been bad in some of my classes. They're worse this year than they were last year. Seems like every time I start some-thing new, like high school, it takes me a long time to get used to it. Sometimes I'm just real tired and I don't want to go to school. If I don't feel good in school, I just go down to the office and lay down or tell them

I want to go home. Last year, when I was really, really sick, I got better grades than now. I had a tutor, but he only came over once a week. I want to go to college, so I got to do better next year. I think I just started on a bad foot. I have to go to summer school. But I'm going to basketball and cancer camp, too.

Sometimes I think the chemotherapy drugs have a big effect on my energy. I'm on maintenance now, so I'm taking 6-MP, Septra, methotrexate. I take them every day in pills. I'm off the prednisone now, but I have to take that five days every month.

The doctor gave me another spinal tap and she said she found abnormal cells and that I have to keep having spinal taps. It doesn't really worry me, but it upset me at first. I think I've got it in control. Maybe there were some bad cells around my back, but not in the rest of my body. I think they can just give me more medicine. I don't think I have to start the whole program over again.

I had to have a spinal tap last week. I was real mad at my mom, so I was uptight for it. It took the doctor a long time to get the needle in my back. It hurt a lot. It was the first time I ever cried from a spinal tap. I was feeling real frustrated. It made it hard on the doctor.

I'm kind of frustrated a lot lately. Sometimes I take it out on my mom, even if it's not her fault. I take a whole lot of medicine, and it makes me feel moody. I get angry. I get mad at my mom when she puts me on punishment and doesn't let me go to work. I don't understand that. I mean, it takes, like, six hours out of the week. That's it. I get paid ten dollars a week for my chores. If I don't do my chores, I don't have no money. My job gives me my own money. It's only two days! I can do my homework.

I work at a youth center. We give dances and stuff, and we help young people stop violence, and we try to give them better things to do than fighting. We get together and talk about problems and go places and have parties. We all have our little fun, and I enjoy doing that. My girlfriend works there. Her aunt talked to us about what we wanted to do in life and everything, and how we feel about certain things. It was good because it got us thinking. It's a good program.

Last week my girlfriend and I had a fight. I came home mad. My mom said that when I get my way I'm OK, but when I don't, look out. She didn't want me to go to work last week because she said I had an attitude. It's not that, it's just that I'm upset by all of this. For a while, my girlfriend and I weren't getting along. Lots of things going through my mind. A lot of

101

pressure. It's kind of hard when I'm not getting good grades. I'm going to have to take things over. My girlfriend doesn't pressure me; she accepts me. I get along with all my friends, like always. Being sick hasn't changed anything. Me and Jimmy are still good friends. We went to Great America last weekend. We had fun.

If I have to start the cancer treatments over again, I'd be upset. I don't think I could go through that again. I don't want to lose my hair. That was really hard. And getting my stomach fat from the steroids. I never throw up or anything from the drugs. A couple of times I'd feel nauseous, but not much. Sometimes, I still wish my Port-a-Cath [vein implant] was in. It was real quick, real easy. With the Port it was no problem. It doesn't make much of a difference without it, but it was easier.

Because of the cancer, I can't really do the same things. If I didn't have my knee problems I could play basketball, but I need to get my wind back up. I can still swim in the lake and go running around it to get myself in shape for camp. Me and Jimmy are going to cancer camp. I'm really looking forward to that. We had fun last year. My girlfriend writes me letters. I write her, too. We keep them in boxes. She said sometimes she hangs my letters on her wall. Most of the time I make up the stuff I write. I've got to fill up the page.

A lot of people can't even stand the word "needle." I'm not scared of that stuff. And I'm not afraid of no doctor. Even if I didn't have nice doctors I wouldn't be scared. I don't really ask them questions 'cause they'll tell me if something is wrong. Like when the doctor called last week to tell me about my cells.

I think everything's going to get better—when I get older, I suppose. Not right now, though. I'm sick. I have treatments for two more years, four years altogether. If I never got that chromosome thing, it would only have been three years of treatment. The doctor said I would be finished when I was 17 or 18 years old. It's not such a long time because the maintenance will stop in about a year, probably, then they just check me once in a while. For now, every two months I get a spinal tap. Except now, since they've got to watch my fluids from the bad cells. After a while, I'll only have to go in every six months or so. I guess I'm lucky I take it so well. Mentally, I think I'm older than most other kids. I've been through stuff even adults haven't been through.

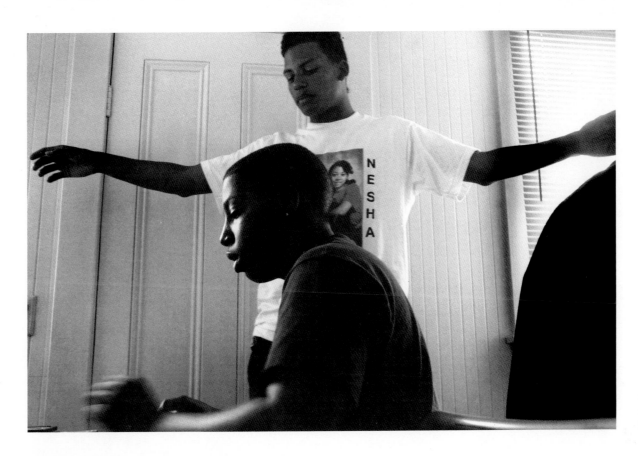

Antione
(sitting) and a
friend.

Update

Antione is feeling good despite a recent recurrence of his cancer. He is continuing his treatments, attending summer school, going to camp, and staying very active. He is in the midst of treatment for the recurrence, which will require an additional three to four years of treatment.

Jimmy has completed his treatment program and is feeling great. He will be going with Antione to a special camp for kids who have cancer or are in remission. Jimmy is looking forward to finishing high school without interruption.

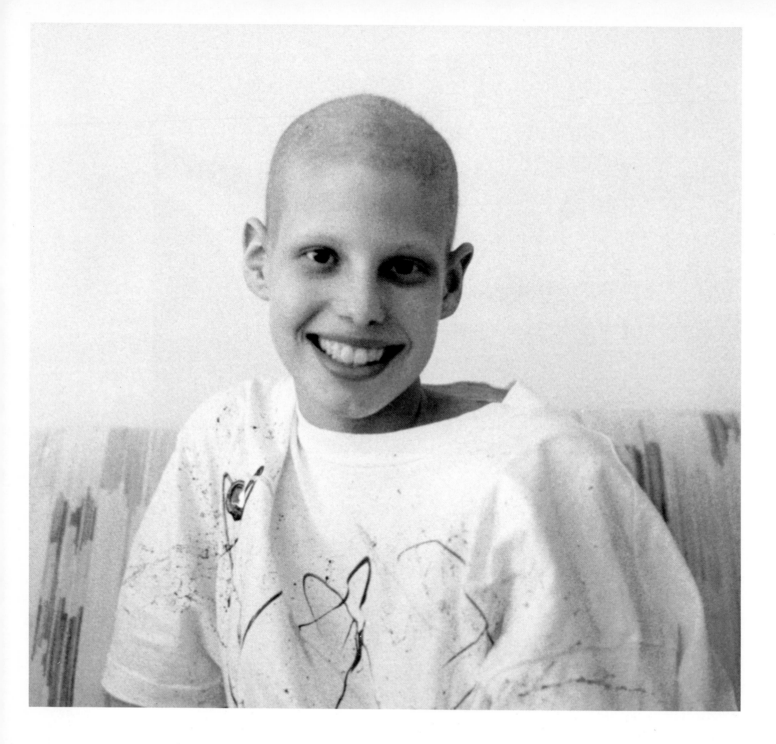

Amanda

15 years old
Osteogenic sarcoma, cancer of the bone

Amanda had been receiving chemotherapy for about eight months when I first meet her. The cancer treatment is very successful, and she is nearing the end of her treatments. Amanda underwent many surgeries during the first few months of her chemotherapy and had a total metal knee replacement, which left a scar running the length of her thigh.

When we sit down to talk, Amanda appears very fragile. However, I soon see that she possesses a tremendous amount of energy in the way she speaks about her disease and the effect it has on her life, her family, and her friends. During our long afternoon visit, we are joined by her mother.

April 1988

Amanda
Fran, Amanda's mother

What were the events that led up to your diagnosis?

Amanda: All along I knew I had something there. I kept asking the doctor, "Are you sure it's not the C-word?" He gave me a brace to keep my leg straight, but it started swelling and I couldn't walk on it. One day the doctor called and my parents were away. I was home watching a scary movie with my friend, and as soon as the phone rang I knew it was bad news. He didn't tell me what was wrong, but he said, "You can tell your parents to come to my office tomorrow morning without an appointment, and you don't have to come." After that I nearly went crazy.

I always had the feeling that one day something was going to happen to me. I felt this cancer all along. My mother didn't tell me what the doctor had told her. All she said was that we had to go see another doctor. I kept saying, "It's the C-word. I know it is."

I have bone cancer. It was in my knee, but now it's all out. When I had my first operation, they found 100 percent kill. That means that before they went into my leg, the cancer was already dead. During this operation the doctors also had to go into my lungs to see if the cancer had traveled there. That's the first place bone cancer goes to if it spreads. Luckily, they didn't find anything in my lungs. It was horrible having both operations within weeks of each other.

Fran: Before we found out Amanda had cancer, we just thought she had pulled a muscle. We went to the hospital, and the doctor did every test possible. He didn't miss a thing, he was great. Nothing showed up, so they did a CAT scan. The only thing she couldn't do was bend her leg all the way. We didn't know what was wrong.

After the doctor told us the news, he told us about different hospitals we could choose. He suggested a cancer hospital, but I thought to myself, "Amanda doesn't need that hospital, she doesn't have cancer." I came home like a crazy person. I called different doctors and got rude secretaries or appointments that were too far away. Finally, I did call the hospital he had recommended, and they were the complete opposite from everyone I'd talked to. The nurse told me to bring Amanda in the next day, and if we had to sit in the waiting room and wait, then that's what we should do. That's what we did, and that's where we ended up.

Amanda: The doctor just looked at the CAT scan, then looked at my leg, and said, "That's it. Just go out to lunch, come back in an hour, and we'll put you in the hospital."

Fran: Amanda had everything done at a hospital in New York. They were wonderful there because they do so much for the kids and families. I got so sick when I first walked in there, but now it's like home away from home. Everyone knows us, they welcome us back. They come running to see Amanda. I'll tell you, it helps. The hospital had a whole day devoted to the siblings of kids who are sick. Amanda's sister, Melanie, got a tour of the chemotherapy room, the operating room, the radiation room, they showed her everything.

Amanda: Melanie knows a little of what I go through, but they showed her stuff she had never seen. They showed her what it's like to put in a Broviac. She said it looked so real, even though it was done on a dummy.

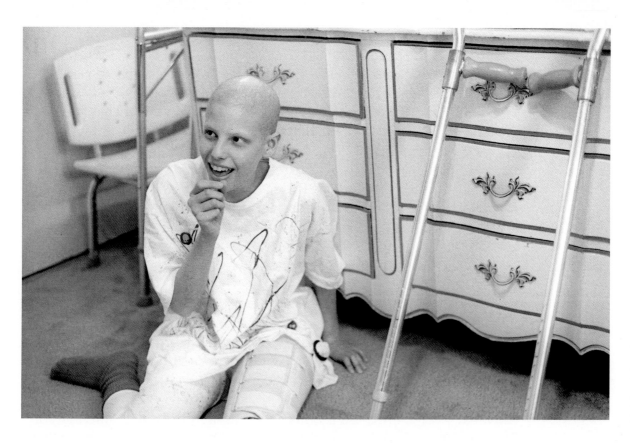

Amanda recovers from her surgery for a total metal knee replacement.

Now I only have five treatments left. Sometimes I get very sick from the chemotherapy. They give me antimedics, which are supposed to help the nausea, but they make me feel weird. They make me very nervous and stuffy, like I can't breathe. I get headaches sometimes, too.

My drugs are methotrexate, vincristine, Bleomycin, Cytoxan, actinomycin D, and adriamycin. I get them as an outpatient, which means that I go into the clinic in the morning, get the medicine, and go home that afternoon. Sometimes I have to go back four days a week, sometimes two. They give me the adriamycin in a pump. It's kind of like wearing a radio, and I can be at home when I get that.

My vein implant makes it pretty easy to get the medication. I've had two put in. The first one was always a problem, and they were never able to draw blood out of it, so I got stuck with needles anyway. But this one, thank God, is much better. They can do anything with it. They give me medicine and take blood from it. Before the Broviac, when they would inject the chemo through my veins, it would sometimes burn me. That doesn't happen now.

107

I mostly always come home after a treatment. A couple of times I had to stay in the hospital because of fevers and infections. So far though, everything's been smooth. I meet a lot of kids through the outpatient clinic. I also meet people when I have to stay in overnight. We talk about being sick. I was in the hospital for seven weeks when I had the knee and the lung operation, and when they put the Broviac in. I also have to have physical therapy on my knee because it isn't bending too well.

Fran: Most of the other parents I've met in the hospital are great. We stay overnight together in the lounge. We play cards, we get a late-night poker game going. We all help each other out. Sometimes though, it feels like parents are in competition with each other. One woman said to me, "Oh, Amanda's not bending her knee as well as my daughter. My daughter can bend her leg all the way now."

Each doctor has his own way of doing things. One kid is running, the other kid is crawling. I know Amanda sometimes gets jealous if someone is doing better, but it shouldn't be a competition. If she limps, she limps. She still has her leg. I mean, if you're not so pretty, you put a little makeup on and you're gorgeous, that's all.

Amanda: Most of my close friends have been great through this, except for one of them, Lisa. I don't know what happened. It really hurts me that she can't be close to me 'cause I'm sick. I've always been a good friend to her. I guess she's scared. We've always been best friends, but in the beginning, she didn't call me at all. Even her little brother, who is only 8, got crazy and started acting abnormal with me. Then Lisa started calling me again, but now she's always with my sister. They do everything together now. That makes me crazy 'cause she's my age, not my sister's.

Fran: I'll tell you, the word "cancer" is a very frightening word. Cancer? Children don't get cancer. Only old people get cancer. But here we're talking about a 16-year-old girl, and all of a sudden her best friend has cancer. Even Amanda couldn't say the word. She's afraid. Lisa couldn't even look Amanda in the eye. She's not afraid she's going to catch it, she's just unable to accept it. Lisa probably wonders how her best friend could get this terrible disease. She's not supposed to have it, she's too young. Lisa shied away, and she doesn't know how to act around Amanda.

Amanda: The day I found out, I called Lisa and just cried on the phone. I think that scared her. I have another friend, Ann, who is great. She calls me every day. She's with the "in" crowd, and I've met a lot of people through her. A lot of my other friends call me every day, and I see them a few times a month. They talk to me, and I tell them everything that's going on. They ask me questions because they want to know. They don't make cancer the only thing we talk about. We talk about what's going on in their lives, too.

At school, in the beginning of the year, my friends said the teachers kept calling my name. They tried to tell the teachers that I wasn't coming in, that I was getting home tutoring. Then the Board of Education called, and we told them the story.

Everyone asks, "Where's Amanda?" My friend Ann just tells them I had an operation; I hurt my knee. When I see people in the street and they ask what's happened, I tell them I've had a skiing accident!

What's been the hardest for you since you were diagnosed?

Amanda: The chemotherapy. The lung operation was also really bad, I couldn't breathe. I couldn't move my leg because I'd recently had the knee operation, and I couldn't move my arm because the Broviac had been put in.

Now, when I'm not getting chemo, I cough a lot, I get mouth sores, fevers, my blood counts drop, I lose a lot of weight. Altogether, I've lost almost twenty pounds. Now, when I have a few weeks off in between treatments, I feel a little more normal and go places. I eat like an animal and try to build my blood counts back up.

Fran: When Amanda is feeling good, she wants to go back to school to visit her old teachers. They call her, they come to the house, they write letters.

Amanda: My sister goes to the same school as I do. She brings the letters back and forth. I had a teacher whose father just died of cancer. We wrote to each other a lot about that. I helped him and he helped me. We had a lot in common. When I came walking into school, he couldn't believe it was me, that I was the same person. I'd changed so much.

Fran: Everyone in the family has been so supportive, so great—my husband, my parents, my sister, my brother. We're very lucky to have such good friends and family. Everyone showed their true colors and came together.

What do you like to do with your free time when you're not in the hospital?

Amanda: Sometimes I stay home and my friends come over. I just really started walking again, and I still use crutches and the leg brace. I'm more steady now than I ever was before. I've been out a few times to eat or to my family's house, but nothing exciting yet. I love going to my aunt's house. She always makes time for me, and her kids are great. She has three boys; I love them and they love me. They are like my own kids. When I was diagnosed, the youngest was only a year old. He had just started walking, and he hopped around trying to copy me! It was the funniest thing. He used to play drums on my bald head. I like going there because it's normal.

Sometimes, when I go shopping with my friends, I count the times people stare at me because I'm bald. It bothers me, but when they stare, I just stare back. I just got a new wig. I have three or four. I also have a hat with a brim so you can't really see anything. I don't like wearing things on my head at home. I hope my hair comes back in time for school. I don't care if it's short, I just want enough to cover my head.

Fran: I feel like I've changed a lot since all of this began. I know more. Now, when someone asks me what they can do, I tell them to write out a check or drop some money to the Ronald McDonald House. That's better than the flowers, the candy. When it all began, I didn't want to be around anybody—not my husband, not my mother, nobody. I would just find a quiet corner in the hospital and sit. I couldn't believe it. One day here we are, such a happy family, and all of a sudden this had to come out. I would cry and say, "Why? Why Amanda?"

A few weeks ago I went away for the weekend. It was the first time I'd been away since Amanda got sick. Everyone told me I should go, that I deserved it. I felt so guilty. How could I go? It turned out to be great. We went to the movies, we listened to music. Everyone needs a little time away.

Amanda: I think this has been very hard on my mother. After my surgery I remember when the doctors came in and told me I had osteogenic sarcoma. I asked, "Well, is it cancer?" I asked if I was going to die; and the doctor said no. I asked a million questions. I get angry about it sometimes and I cry. I'll be watching TV or something, and out of nowhere I'll start to cry. Still though, I've made it this far, and it's almost over.

In the beginning, when you're first diagnosed, they see how bad you are and they put you on a certain protocol. I got six weeks of chemotherapy right away. The higher the kill, the fewer drugs you have to take. My friends ask me which drug is the worst. I think they're all pretty bad. I don't tell the other kids in the hospital that the doctors were very positive about my recovery from the beginning because most of them are not lucky enough to have that. I don't want to make anyone feel bad. I don't brag about it.

Fran: People would come into the room when Amanda was in the hospital and ask how she was doing. Even if Amanda was sick as a dog, I'd say, "Fine, thank you," or "She's had better days." One woman whose son was diagnosed at the same time Amanda was said to me, "You know Fran, you're the only one in this room who can say 'fine' and really mean it." I said to her, "You know, I want to tell you something. What do you want me to do? I wish your son were doing as well as Amanda." People ask me how she is. What should I say? There shouldn't be such insensitivity.

Did you meet young people in the hospital who later died?

Amanda: Yeah. But I don't know their names, just their faces. I never wanted to be around the other sick people. I always wanted to be alone or with my roommate. I never wanted to leave my room, even when the volunteers asked me to go to the playroom. After a while I did go to the playroom, and I liked it. I guess I didn't go before because I was scared. I knew everyone would be bald. I didn't want to look around. It was traumatic for me. The first time I went into the hospital I covered my eyes until I got to my room. I didn't want to see. These were things I'd never seen before. I feel positive about my recovery now. I don't remember much from the beginning, but I'm sure I had my doubts.

Fran: I remember after the doctors looked at her, the whole family was in the room. I said, "We're all going to hold hands. We're going to form a chain, and this chain will never, never be broken. We're a family. We're in it together. She suffers, we all suffer. We're going to lick this. There is a team of doctors out there, but we're the stronger team, and we're going to do it." I've never been a religious person, but when people would call and say they would say a prayer for her, I would say, "Please do. Please do."

April 1988

Amanda and Ann have been close friends for several years. Ann comes over to see Amanda frequently, and they share their deepest secrets. Ann stopped by during our visit, and joins in the conversation.

Amanda
Ann, Amanda's best friend

How do you feel about your best friend having cancer?

Ann: Amanda hasn't changed. She seems stronger. A lot of other kids ask me about her, how she's doing. They always tell me they feel bad when they haven't called her. I say they should call, but I guess some of them feel weird. I never ever feel funny around her. Amanda's my best friend.

    I'm the type of person who accepts things for what they are. Sometimes I still don't believe it. You never expect this to happen to someone so close to you or so young. Through this, I've learned how good a friend I can be. I would never have known until something like this happened. I always knew that Amanda would always be Amanda. She's still the same. Her body's physically sick, but that's about it. I couldn't believe how much weight she's lost. One day, all of a sudden, she's skin and bones.

Amanda: Ann's been great to me. If we can't see each other, she at least calls. It really hurts me that Lisa can't be close to me because I've got

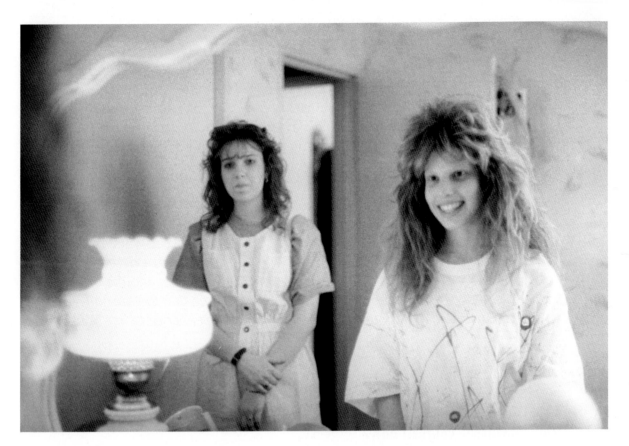

Amanda shows off one of her wigs to her friend Ann.

cancer. When she had hepatitis I called her all the time, I went up to her house. It hurt me so much because I was such a good friend.

Ann: Even in the dead of winter I come over. I live two blocks away. Lisa lives right in this building, so there's no reason she can't come up. I mean, I'm here two, three times a week, every single week. It makes me angry that Lisa stays away.

Amanda: I don't ask why I got cancer. I know there is no answer. I've always been a sissy. I never smoked, and I only took little sips of my parents' drinks. I see kids who smoke pot at parties, but I didn't. I was always good. I always took care of myself. If all goes well, I should be finished with my treatments this June. I can't wait for that day.

113

June 1991

Three years after our first meeting, I visit Amanda in New York. She and her boyfriend pick me up at the train station, and we go for a ride, skirting the amusements at Coney Island. We have a great afternoon talking and catching up on one another's lives. After her boyfriend goes home, we drive back to Amanda's house and sit down to talk about her life since recovering from cancer.

Amanda tells me about her life as a physical-therapy student in her second year at Brooklyn College. She readily acknowleges that she might never have had an interest in physical therapy if not for her own success with her recovery. She shows me photographs of herself when she was in the hospital, during her operations, and when she received treatments. It is hard to believe that the young woman in front of me, and the one in the pictures, are the same person. She also shows me that the scar on her leg remains, and occasionally she limps, a lifetime reminder of her bout with cancer.

Amanda

How do you see yourself now?

I look at life more seriously now. I'm more mature. When I think of all the drugs that have gone through my body for cancer treatment, I would never do drugs to get high. I hate when anyone is prejudiced against sick people or makes fun of them. Having cancer has affected everything I do now. I would never have thought about going into physical therapy. My life would have taken another direction. I look back on the pictures from when I was sick, and I can't hate them. It was my life. What could I do about it? I had to accept it. Luckily, I'm fine now.

How is your leg and your general health?

From the middle of my thigh to the middle of my calf, it is all metal. They took the bone out. I have a hinge where the kneecap was. The metal is cemented into the rest of the bone. All the muscle around the scar is

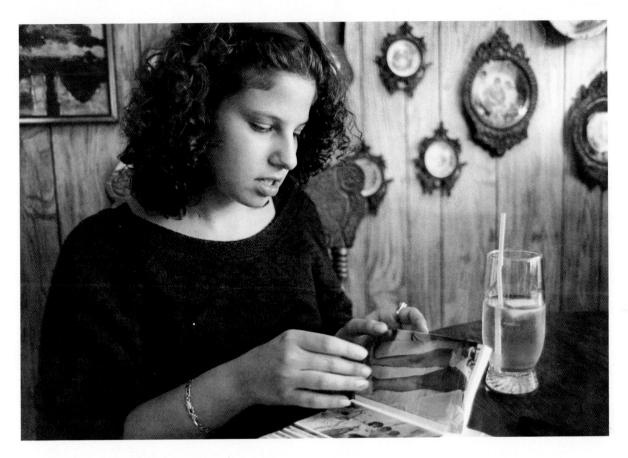

Now in good health, Amanda looks at photos of herself when she was sick and in the hospital.

dead now. Sometimes it bothers me to look at the pictures of myself then, especially because I was so thin.

I remember how good it felt when my leg finally touched the ground. I'd spent so much time in bed in the hospital. Once, a whole glass IV bottle fell on me when I was in bed, right after my lung operation. The bottle broke all over me, and I couldn't move, I was still hooked up to a machine. A tube an inch thick was coming out of me, so I couldn't scream. It was awful. I thought I was going to die. I thought my mother was going to kill the nurse.

Now, three years after I'm out of treatment, I still go back to the hospital for checkups every three months. It's hard not to get freaked out and think that they're going to tell me something is wrong. Every year that passes, I go another month in between checkups. It's like a regular doctor's appointment.

Looking back, how do you view the time you were sick?

It was terrible, especially the chemotherapy. Even now, I can't go back to the outpatient clinic where I got the medicine. I get nauseous even thinking about it. I remember the smell, the blue room. I can't drink the water. I can't use the lotion. I hate it.

A couple of times I had to talk to people who were just diagnosed with cancer. I told them I wasn't going to lie, the whole thing is terrible. I said, "It might not be as bad for you as it was for me, but nobody can tell you that it's easy. It's the hardest thing in the world. I don't think there is anything harder than getting through cancer."

How do you view your health now?

I'm thankful. Whenever I get the chance to wish for anything, I always wish that my health stays good. I'm very emotional, especially when anyone dies. I still can't believe things like this could have happened to me, or anyone else I know.

Sometimes out of the blue, a word or something will make me remember that I once had cancer. I don't think of the specifics, I just think of it in general. I always think to myself that nobody now would ever believe that I was so sick. Like, a lot of people at work ask me why I have this scar running down my leg, or why I've started to limp. When I tell them, they are all really nice about it.

I feel totally normal now, except this winter when I couldn't go skiing with my friends. That pissed me off. What was I going to do, sit in the car? My boyfriend would like to go skating with me, but I can't do that either. He's good about it, but I wish I could go with him. The problem is, I don't have the muscle in my upper thigh.

My family still makes me crazy sometimes. They always ask how my leg is. It's like everybody else's leg, you know? They baby me some, like my grandparents and my father. Sometimes all the attention gets to me. It's still like when I was sick. I don't need it now. I get worried that when I have kids, I won't be able to run after them. Maybe I'll have another operation by then.

Eventually, they want to take muscle out of my back and put it in my leg. I've seen the scar the operation leaves, and it's disgusting. I don't

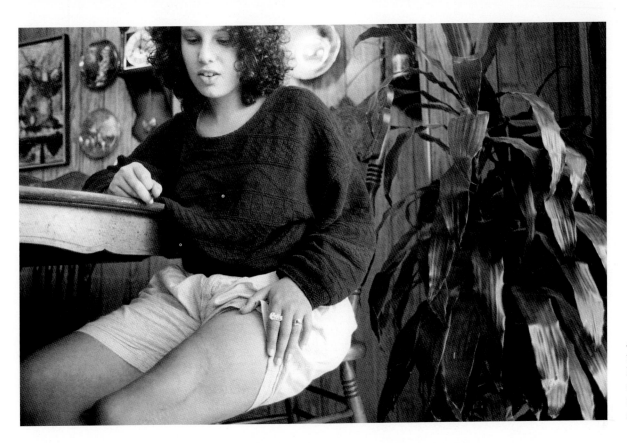

Amanda shows the scar on her leg, a reminder of her cancer treatment and surgery.

really care, I mean, who do I have to impress? I just don't want to go through the surgery again. It all still feels pretty recent.

Do you feel like you've had an influence on anyone in your life?

Yeah, on my friend Lisa, the one who I wasn't close to when I was sick. Now we are good friends again, and she's sorry that we weren't friends when I was sick. Also my boyfriend, but I still haven't let him see the pictures of me from when I was getting chemotherapy. We always talk about it, though.

That girl Ann, the one who I was good friends with before, is out of my life now. She thought I was going with her boyfriend behind her back. She picked him over me. I've given her chances, but she's messed them up. I know I've had an influence on her life. She always tells people that she has a friend named Amanda. I know she still loves me. She was with me through everything. A part of me does love Ann because she was always there for me when I was sick.

Ann wrote me this letter:

> . . . *Last year when you were sick I was able to share absolutely everything with you, I wanted to make you a part of everything. Sometimes I think you don't need me anymore. I don't know if I'm insulting you or what, I just have to get this out in the open. I feel that last year you needed someone to keep you strong. I was that someone. Now I feel you don't need me or my strength anymore.*
>
> *Don't you dare think I was there for you when you were sick out of pity. I didn't have to be there for you. I chose to be. I chose to spend all those afternoons and nights with you. What did I get out of it? I didn't get a good deed award. I didn't get a promise from God that I'd go to heaven. I got your friendship, which was more than I could have asked for. I'm sorry for the way I've been recently. I value your friendship more than anyone else's. We have been through so much good and bad together. I thought our friendship was so strong. I never thought anything could get in our way.*

I think that positive thinking had a lot to do with my getting better. I didn't want to die. All my life I've wanted to have kids. I just looked forward to that, and having a boyfriend. I was 15 when I got cancer. I was thinking of the things teenage girls think of. I had all my friends, and my cousins, too. They helped me. I wanted to be around for all of them.

Update

Amanda continues to have good health and she can do most activities with her leg with few exceptions. She has changed her college major from physical therapy to general health.

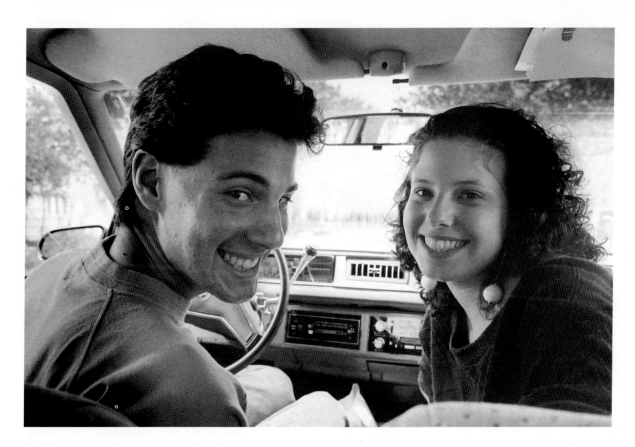

Amanda and
her boyfriend,
whom she met
shortly after
completing her
cancer therapy.

Glossary

ANEMIA: A decrease in the hemoglobin content of circulating red blood cells.

ANESTHESIOLOGIST: A doctor specializing in anesthesia. His or her duties include prescribing the drugs and method of anesthesia.

ANESTHETIC: A chemical agent that prevents pain when injected or inhaled.

ANGIOGRAPHY: An X-ray study of the blood or lymph vessels that requires a patient to be injected with an opaque dye.

ANTIBIOTIC: A chemical substance that is able to stop the growth of other micro-organisms, especially bacteria. Antibiotics are used mainly for the treatment of bacterial infections.

ANTIBODY: A protein developed by the body that helps defend the body against infection. When foreign organisms appear in the blood or tissues, antibodies are produced to neutralize them.

ANTIEMETIC: A drug, such as zofran, that prevents or alleviates nausea and vomiting.

BACTERIA: A term for a group of living organisms, larger than viruses, that may be seen only through a microscope. While many bacteria live peacefully in normal, healthy bodies, some bacteria can cause infections.

BENIGN TUMOR: A noncancerous (nonmalignant) growth that does not metastasize or spread to other body sites.

BIOPSY: The removal of cells or tissue for microscopic examination. Biopsies are performed through an incision or by a needle.

BLAST CELL: An immature white blood cell. Normally, the bone marrow consists of less than 5 percent blasts. When a child has leukemia these abnormal cells multiply rapidly and crowd out the normal blood cells in the body.

BLOOD TRANSFUSION: The administration of red blood cells, usually from someone else.

BONE MARROW ASPIRATION: Marrow is the red spongy material inside large bone cavities that manufactures blood cells. To test the condition of marrow, doctors remove a sample from a bone in the chest, hip, spine, or leg through a suction needle.

BONE MARROW TRANSPLANT: A procedure that replaces a patient's destroyed marrow with healthy marrow. The new marrow is harvested either from a donor or from the patient's own marrow during remission. The marrow is then frozen and is later reinfused.

CANCER: An out-of-control and aimless growth of cells that can spread beyond its site of origin.

CARCINOGEN: A substance that causes cancer.

CARDIAC: Pertaining to the heart.

Catheter: A hollow tube used for injection and withdrawal of fluids. A catheter can be made of rubber, plastic, glass, or metal.

Chemotherapy: A method of cancer treatment that uses chemical agents or drugs to destroy malignant cells.

Complete blood count (CBC): Examination of the blood to determine the quantity of red and white blood cells and platelets.

Computerized tomographic scan (CT scan or CAT scan): An X ray using special computers that make cross-sectional pictures of the body and shows details not seen on conventional X rays.

Dehydration: Excessive loss of fluids from the body.

Diuretic: A drug that increases the body's ability to eliminate urine.

Echocardiogram: An imaging technique that uses sound waves to visualize the heart in motion.

Electrocardiography (EKG, ECG): A painless test that graphically records the heart's rate, rhythm, and spatial orientation. Disc-shaped conductors called electrodes are attached to the body. Then an apparatus called an electrocardiograph amplifies and traces on paper the heart's minute electrical impulses.

Electroencephalography (EEG): A test that records electrical activity in the brain. Electrodes are affixed to the skull with paste. Then an electroencephalograph records the electrical impulses as brain waves. Abnormal wave patterns suggest a possible malignancy or other diseases or damage.

Endoscopy: A medical procedure in which a doctor inserts a flexible tubular instrument called an endoscope through the mouth, nose, or anus to examine body cavities and hollow organs.

Finger stick: A blood-testing procedure in which a few drops of blood are taken from a fingertip that has been pricked with a sharp needle.

Gallium scan: A type of nuclear scan in which the patient is injected with a radioactive material called gallium-67. Over several days, the material localizes in sites of inflammation, including cancerous lymph nodes and other tumors. When the body is subsequently scanned, the sites of inflammation are identified.

Gastrointestinal tract (GI): The digestive tract, which includes the esophagus, stomach, and intestines.

Graft: A surgical procedure in which healthy bone, skin, or other tissue replaces diseased, damaged, or amputated parts of the body.

Hematology: The study of the blood and blood-forming organs and their diseases.

HEMATOMA: Blood or fluid that has seeped out of a vein and collected in an organ, space, or tissue, causing pain, swelling, or inflammation.

HEMOGLOBIN: A compound of protein and iron contained within the red blood cells. Oxygen is carried from the lungs to the tissues of the body in hemoglobin. It also transports carbon dioxide, a waste product, from the tissues to the lungs, to be exhaled.

HEMORRHAGE: Loss of blood, either externally or internally, caused by injury to the blood vessel walls or by a deficiency of certain blood clotting elements such as platelets.

HODGKIN'S DISEASE: The most common lymphatic-system cancer, Hodgkin's disease is found mostly in young people between the ages of 15 and 34. Hodgkin's disease generally responds very well to treatment.

HORMONE THERAPY: Cancer treatment by chemical supplementation or blockage of hormones.

HYPERGLYCEMIA: Abnormally increased content of sugar in the blood.

HYPOGLYCEMIA: Abnormally decreased content of sugar in the blood.

INFLAMMATION: A local response to cell injury characterized by redness, heat, pain, swelling, and loss of function. Inflammation serves to destroy, dilute, or wall off the source of injury and the injured tissue.

INTRAVENOUS (IV): Administering drugs, blood products, or fluids directly into a vein, either through infusion (IV drip) or injection (IV needle). Drugs can also be injected intramuscularly (into the muscle tissue), subcutaneously (just beneath the skin's surface), intra-arterially (into an artery), intracavitarily (into the abdomen or the lung's pleural cavity), or intrathecally (into the spinal fluid).

JAUNDICE: A yellowish discoloration of the skin and the white portion of the eyes due to the accumulation of bilirubin, a product of hemoglobin breakdown. Jaundice is usually caused by liver disease or an abnormally rapid breakdown of red blood cells.

LEUKEMIA: The most common childhood malignancy. Leukemia is cancer of the blood and blood-producing tissue, especially the bone marrow. Acute lymphocytic leukemia (ALL) accounts for 85 percent of all childhood leukemia cases. Other forms of acute leukemia include acute nonlymphocytic leukemias (ANLL), which consist of acute myelocytic leukemia, acute monocytic leukemia, acute promyelocytic leukemia, erythroleukemia, and myelomonocytic leukemia. The chronic leukemias include chronic myelogenous leukemia, and chronic lymphocytic leukemia, which does not occur in children.

LOCALIZED CANCER: A malignancy found only in the original (primary) site.

Lumbar puncture (spinal tap): Diagnostic procedure in which spinal fluid is withdrawn from the lower spinal area with a needle.

Lymph: A clear yellowish fluid consisting primarily of white blood cells called lymphocytes. Lymph travels through the lymphatic system, bathing body tissues to help combat infection.

Lymph nodes: Bean-shaped organs that filter bacteria, viruses, dead cells, and other harmful agents from the lymphatic system. They are distributed throughout the body. With infection or cancer, lymph nodes may become infected or enlarged.

Lymphoma: Cancer of the lymphatic system. There are several types of non-Hodgkin's lymphomas. Hodgkin's disease is quite different and is probably not a lymphoma although it is often categorized as such.

Magnetic resonance imaging (MRI): A relatively new, noninvasive imaging technique, similar to a CAT scan, which creates cross-sectional pictures of the body by means of a powerful magnet linked to a computer.

Maintenance therapy: In the state of remission, there are no cancer cells visible anywhere in the body. However, there still may be cancer cells in numbers too small to be visible. Maintenance therapy is aimed at getting rid of these few remaining cells.

Malignant tumor: A cancerous tumor capable of metastasizing.

Metastasis: The spread of cancer from its original site.

Myelogram: A test in which X-ray dye is injected after a lumbar puncture. This test shows whether there is compression of the spinal cord by a tumor.

Neoplasm: Any new or uncontrolled growth, benign or malignant, of abnormal tissue or tumor.

Neurologist: A physician specializing in diseases of the nervous system.

Neutrophils (polys or segs): Granular white blood cells that play a major role in the body's defense against bacteria.

Nuclear scan (radioisotope studies): An imaging technique in which the patient swallows or is injected with a harmless radioactive material that localizes in certain tissues or organs. Electronic devices then track through this material, and the images help physicians determine whether or not organs such as kidneys, liver, and brain are functioning properly. These scans expose patients to less radiation than regular X rays.

Oncology: The branch of medicine dealing with the origin, cause, growth, and treatment of cancer.

PATHOLOGIST: A doctor specializing in identifying diseases through microscopic study.

PLASMA: The liquid portion of the blood in which the blood cells are suspended. Plasma also contains many proteins and minerals necessary for normal body functioning.

PLATELETS: Particles in the blood that aid in blood clotting and act to prevent bleeding.

PROGNOSIS: A prediction of a disease's likely outcome; an assessment of the patient's chances for recovery.

PROPHYLACTIC: Treatment designed to prevent a disease or complication that has not yet developed.

PROTOCOL: A standardized, detailed treatment program for a particular type of cancer.

RADIATION THERAPY: A method of cancer treatment that uses penetrating rays to damage tumor cells. In the process, normal cells are injured also, although they are less likely to die. The aim of the treatment is to injure the tumor cells so they cannot repair or reproduce and will die. Radiation therapy is used by itself or in conjunction with chemotherapy and surgery.

RADIOLOGIST: A physician trained in radiology, the science of interpreting medical X rays.

REGRESSION: A return to a previous state. In cancer, regression occurs when tumors shrink or disappear.

REINDUCTION: The process of starting treatment again after the recurrence of disease.

RELAPSE: The reappearance of cancer after a period during which the initial cancer had abated or disappeared.

REMISSION: Temporary or permanent condition in which no cancer is detected, though cancerous cells may remain in the body in small numbers. At that point, patients are said to be "in remission."

SARCOMA: A malignant tumor that originates in the bones, cartilage, muscle, or blood vessels. Sarcomas often metastasize by way of the bloodstream and grow rapidly.

STAGING: A classification system used by doctors for identifying the extent of the disease.

SYSTEMIC TREATMENT: Cancer therapy, such as chemotherapy, that affects cells throughout the body.

TOXICITY: The harmful side effects caused by a drug.

TUMOR: Any abnormal growth or mass.

URINALYSIS: Examination of urine.

VIRUSES: A group of microorganisms smaller than bacteria that can produce disease. Common viral infections include measles, mumps, chicken pox, and the common cold.

X RAYS: High-energy electromagnetic radiation used in low dosages to "photograph" the inner body and in high dosages to treat cancer.

Chemotherapy Drugs

ACTINOMYCIN-D: Administered by intravenous injection to patients with Wilms' tumor, rhabdomyosarcoma, and bone sarcomas. Some side effects may include mouth and lip sores, hair loss, nausea or vomiting, or low blood counts.

ADRIAMYCIN (DOXORUBICIN): Administered by IV injection to patients with acute leukemia, Wilms' tumor, neuroblastoma, soft-tissue sarcomas, bone sarcomas, Hodgkin's disease, non-Hodgkin's lymphomas, and brain tumors. Side effects may include nausea and vomiting, heart palpitations, pain at the site of injection, fever, chills, sore throat, itchy skin, hair loss, and low blood counts.

ARA-C (CYTOSINE ARABINOSIDE): Administered by injection to patients with acute leukemia. Some side effects may include fever, chills, unusual bleeding or bruising, numbness or tingling in fingers, toes, or face. There may also be mouth and lip sores, general discomfort, nausea, and low blood counts.

ASPARAGINASE: Administered by injection directly into the muscle and occasionally into the vein. Some side effects may include labored breathing, joint pain, swollen ankles, and low blood counts.

BLEOMYCIN: Administered by intravenous or intramuscular injection. Side effects may include fever and chills, coughing, mouth sores, darkening of skin, appetite loss, lung damage, and low blood counts.

CYTOXAN (CYCLOPHOSPHAMIDE): Administered orally or by injection to patients with acute leukemia, Hodgkin's disease, non-Hodgkin's lymphomas, and neuroblastoma. Side effects may include bloody or painful urination, fever, chills, sore throat, mouth and lip sores, darkening of the skin and fingernails, appetite and hair loss, nausea and vomiting, and low blood counts. In teenage girls, there may be missed menstrual periods.

DAUNOMYCIN (DAUNORUBICIN): Administered by intravenous injection to patients with acute leukemia. Side effects may include nausea and vomiting, heart palpitations, pain at the site of injection, fever, chills, sore throat, itchy skin, hair loss, and low blood counts. Reddish urine may result one or two days after the injection.

METHOTREXATE: Administered orally or by injection to patients with acute leukemia, non-Hodgkin's lymphomas, and bone sarcomas. Side effects may include mouth sores, nausea and vomiting, appetite loss, and low blood counts.

PREDNISONE: Administered orally to patients with acute leukemia and non-Hodgkin's lymphomas. Side effects may include depression, mood changes, muscle cramps, extreme fatigue, increased weight gain and appetite, and difficulty sleeping. In teenage girls, there may also be menstrual problems.

6-Mercaptopurine (6-MP): A drug belonging to a group called antimetabolites, which resemble the "building blocks" of DNA. When the cell constructs new DNA it takes up 6-MP by mistake, and the DNA does not work. This drug is taken orally as a single daily dose as part of maintenance therapy for leukemia.

Vincristine: Administered by IV injection to patients with Hodgkin's disease, non-Hodgkin's lymphomas, rhabdomyosarcoma, neuroblastoma, and Wilms' tumor. Some side effects may include blurred or double vision, stomach cramps, constipation, difficulty walking, joint pain, numbness in fingers and toes, seizures, hair and weight loss, and low blood counts.

Methods of Administering Chemotherapy

Broviac-Hickman catheter: A catheter that is surgically implanted into a large vein in the upper chest, where it can remain for up to two years as a permanent IV line. Medicine is fed into the tube's top, which carries it to the veins.

Intramuscularly (IM): Some drugs must seep gradually into the bloodstream to be effective. These are injected into a muscle in the arm, thigh, or buttocks and take no more than several seconds.

Intravenously: The most prevalent and fastest way of introducing chemotherapeutic drugs into the bloodstream is directly through the veins. Doctors either inject the chemicals using a syringe (push), or insert the hollow needle, then infuse the medicine slowly (drip) from a plastic bag hanging from a portable pole. Before chemotherapy takes effect, a liquid sedative and antinausea medicine are frequently given to dull adverse reactions, as are fluids for flushing the drugs through the system.

Orally: Many drugs are available in ingestible liquid, capsule, or tablet form. They enter the blood through the lining of the stomach or upper intestines. Not all anticancer medicines can be taken by mouth because they either damage the stomach lining or aren't readily absorbed.

Glossary compiled by James Tulsky, M.D., and John T. Truman, M.D.

Resources

American Cancer Society
1599 Clifton Road NE
Atlanta, GA 30329
(800) 227-2345 for state headquarters
(404) 320-3333 for national headquarters
As the largest private source of cancer research funds in the United States, the American Cancer Society is dedicated to the elimination of cancer through research, education and prevention, patient services, advocacy, and rehabilitation.

Candlelighters Childhood Cancer Foundation
7910 Woodmont Avenue, Suite 460
Bethesda, MD 20814
(800) 366-2223
Candlelighters supports and advocates for families coping with childhood cancer, provides information on treatment options, and maintains a toll-free hotline and speakers bureau.

Association for the Care of Children's Health
7910 Woodmont Avenue, Suite 300
Bethesda, MD 20814
(301) 654-6549
ACCH promotes family-centered care policies that are responsive to the unique developmental and psychosocial needs of children and their families and brings together a variety of disciplines related to children's health-care issues and services.

National Association of Children's Hospitals and Related Institutions
401 Wythe Street
Alexandria, VA 22314
(703) 684-1355
NACHRI represents children's hospitals throughout the United States and advocates for the improvement of institution-based health-care services for children.

Cancer Information Service
National Institutes of Health
9000 Rockville Pike
Bethesda, MD 20892
(800) 422-6237
CIS is a network of nineteen regional offices providing the most current information on cancer prevention, screening, diagnosis, treatment, and continuing care.

Leukemia Society of America
600 Third Avenue
New York, NY 10016
(800) 955-4572
Through research and education, LSA seeks the cause and eventual cure for leukemia and its related diseases—lymphomas and multiple myeloma.

Ronald McDonald House
500 N. Michigan Avenue, Suite 200
Chicago, IL 60611
(312) 836-7384
More than 150 Ronald McDonald Houses in nine countries provide low-cost, temporary lodging for the families of seriously ill children being treated at nearby hospitals.

Other Titles Available from NewSage Press

Blue Moon over Thurman Street
by Ursula K. Le Guin
Photographs by Roger Dorband

When the Bough Breaks:
Pregnancy and the Legacy of Addiction
by Kira Corser and Frances Payne Adler

Organizing for Our Lives:
New Voices from Rural Communities
by Richard Steven Street and Samuel Orozco
Foreword by Cesar Chavez

The New Americans:
Immigrant Life in Southern California
by Ulli Steltzer

Family Portraits in Changing Times
by Helen Nestor

Stories of Adoption: Loss and Reunion
by Eric Blau

Exposures: Women & Their Art
by Betty Ann Brown and Arlene Raven
Photographs by Kenna Love

A Portrait of American Mothers & Daughters
by Raisa Fastman

Women & Work:
Photographs and Personal Writings
by Maureen R. Michelson
Photographs edited by Michael Dressler &
Maureen R. Michelson

Common Heroes:
Facing a Life Threatening Illness
by Eric Blau

For a complete catalog, write to:
NewSage Press
825 N.E. 20th Ave., Suite 150
Portland, OR 97232
(503) 232-6794